M000299908

RECOVERING

COMPULSIVE

OVEREATER

RECOVERY FROM COMPULSIVE OVEREATING
DAILY MEDITATIONS

BY ANONYMOUS RECOVERING COMPULSIVE OVEREATERS

Recovering Compulsive Overeater
Daily Meditations
By Anonymous Members of Twelve Step Recovery Programs

Cover Illustration: Mercedes McDonald

(c) 2009 All Rights Reserved

Partnerships for Community
561 Hudson Street, Suite 23
New York, N.Y. 10014

Printed in United States

ISBN-13: 978-1-933639-62-8
ISBN-10: 1-933639-62-8

Library of Congress Cataloging-in-Publication Data

Recovering compulsive overeater : daily meditations / by
anonymous members of twelve step recovery programs.
    p. cm.
 ISBN-13: 978-1-933639-62-8
 ISBN-10: 1-933639-62-8
 1. Compulsive behavior--Psychological aspects. 2. Reducing
diet--Psychological aspects. 3. Twelve-step programs-
-Religious aspects--Meditations. 4. Self-care, Health-
-Quotations, maxims, etc. 5. Devotional calendars.
 RC533.R435 2009
 242'.4--dc22
                                    2009020866

PREFACE

Recovering Compulsive Overeater is an inspirational reader used by members of Overeaters Anonymous and others with eating disorders, substance abuse problems, or behavior addictions. Anonymous individuals who practice Twelve Step Recovery decided to produce this daily reader to more fully reflect our experience with dieting and recovery from dieting and compulsive eating. Such collective wisdom helps us to view each day as an opportunity for happiness by focusing on the reality of today without the burdens of compulsive overeating and the diet products and methods we have tried. We are on a brighter firmer path. Our experience with compulsive overeating and the weight loss methods we used is where we first tried to solve life problems. It is where we first hit bottom. Diet remedies and compulsive dieting made us sick and impaired our thinking. We came into Twelve Step Recovery. Health with weight management is possible. These meditations are by and for recovering compulsive overeaters.

With quotes from Anne Lamott, Camryn Manheim, Bob Dylan, Joan Didion, Oprah Winfrey, Alice Walker, Aimee Liu, and other notables, past and present, used in concert with the meditations, this reader brings some of the pleasures and rewards about truth-telling and arriving at self-truth to the surface. Selections deal with our desperation and fear, misconceptions about life, and especially, how our ideas of love, the terrors of love, and romantic addiction have played into our use of diet remedies and methods we have tried. We talk about what we have tried for control, invisibility, buying time, putting off or conquering life. We identify 'So Many Lies' about the remedies, behaviors and methods, and tell about putting our lives on the basis of truth. We tell what happened to make us stop using compulsive dieting and to come into Twelve Step Recovery. We share about "Self-Care" and "Building On Identity" - what we do to practice clear thinking, detach from erroneous messages, clear away self-deception, develop kindness toward self and others, be safe, recognize and deal effectively with attack voices, deal with overwhelming emotions, know and practice courage, serve, and build identity based on our God-given talents, abilities and enthusiasms. We talk about love, honor, loving self, loving another, loving the world.

his daily reader makes reference to the Twelve Steps of Alcoholics Anonymous. It is inspired by the Twelve Steps of Recovery used in Alcoholics Anonymous and Overeaters Anonymous. O.A. uses the Twelve Steps to deal with food. A.A. deals with the Twelve Steps to deal with alcohol. A.A. has granted permission to adapt the Twelve Steps of Alcoholics Anonymous for dealing with compulsive dieting. We add Step 0. Step 0 is the moment of clarity where we realized we could no longer take diet substances or diet compulsively, and that abstinence from compulsive dieting is necessary for us.

e have tried many things: not eating, liquid fasts, appetite suppressants, central nervous system stimulants, diet boosters, diet blasters, diet blockers, metabolizers, diet bitter herbs, diet herbal teas, diet powders, diet liquids, diet pills, diuretics, purging, laxatives, punishing exercise, prescription drugs, over the counter drugs, compulsive exercise or combinations and variations of all of them.

hese selections provide a long-term perspective on the process of living joyously without the compulsions of dieting and eating compulsively. It is possible to refrain from the insane urges we have been smitten with. Health with weight management is possible. We let go of magical thinking. We build on identity. We open up to constructive imagination. We open up to attainable satisfactions.

he anonymous individuals here contribute their own experience, stories, and affirmations. The voices of the individual contributors are their own. The meditations are reinforced by appropriate quotations. The use of these quotes implies no endorsement by the individual quoted or the volumes quoted. These selections contain references to gender, race, and creed, but the ideas and thoughts are applicable to people of all ages, gender, race and creed. This reader is not official conference approved literature of A.A, Overeaters Anonymous, or Greysheeter's Anonymous. If you think you want to let go of diet substances and compulsive dieting, this reader is for you.

 hese meditations are by and for recovering compulsive overeaters.

THE TWELVE STEPS OF
ALCOHOLICS ANONYMOUS

1. We admitted we were powerless over alcohol—that our lives had become unmanageable.

2. Came to believe that a Power greater than ourselves could restore us to sanity.

3. Made a decision to turn our will and our lives over to the care of God as we understood Him.

4. Made a searching and fearless moral inventory of ourselves.

5. Admitted to God, to ourselves, and to another human being the exact nature of our wrongs.

6. Were entirely ready to have God remove all these defects of character.

7. Humbly asked Him to remove our shortcomings.

8. Made a list of all persons we had harmed, and became willing to make amends to them all.

9. Made direct amends to such people wherever possible, except when to do so would injure them or others.

10. Continued to take personal inventory and when we were wrong promptly admitted it.

11. Sought through prayer and meditation to improve our conscious contact with God as we understood Him, praying only for knowledge of His will for us and the power to carry that out.

12. Having had a spiritual awakening as the result of these steps, we tried to carry this message to others, and to practice these principles in all our affairs.

The Twelve Steps and Twelve Traditions of Alcoholics Anonymous have been reprinted and adapted with the permission of Alcoholics Anonymous World Services Inc. ("AAWS"). Permission to reprint and adapt the Twelve Steps and Twelve Traditions does not mean that Alcoholics Anonymous is affiliated with this program. A.A. is a program of recovery from alcoholism only - use of A.A.'s Steps and Traditions or an adapted version of its Steps and Traditions in connection with programs and activities which are patterned after A.A., but which address other problems, or use in any other non-A.A. context, does not imply otherwise. --Alcoholics Anonymous, World Services

THE TWELVE STEPS
ADAPTED FOR COMPULSIVE DIETING

1. We admitted we were powerless over diet substances and compulsive dieting—that our lives had become unmanageable.

2. Came to believe that a Power greater than ourselves could restore us to sanity.

3. Made a decision to turn our will and our lives over to the care of God as we understood Him.

4. Made a searching and fearless moral inventory of ourselves.

5. Admitted to God, to ourselves, and to another human being the exact nature of our wrongs.

6. Were entirely ready to have God remove all these defects of character.

7. Humbly asked Him to remove our shortcomings.

8. Made a list of all persons we had harmed, and became willing to make amends to them all.

9. Made direct amends to such people wherever possible, except when to do so would injure them or others.

10. Continued to take personal inventory and when we were wrong promptly admitted it.

11. Sought through prayer and meditation to improve our conscious contact with God as we understood Him, praying only for knowledge of His will for us and the power to carry that out.

12. Having had a spiritual awakening as the result of these steps, we tried to carry this message to others, and to practice these principles in all our affairs.

Permission to use the Twelve Steps and Twelve Traditions of Alcoholics Anonymous for adaptation granted by A.A. World Services, Inc.

THE TWELVE STEPS OF OVEREATERS ANONYMOUS

1. We admitted we were powerless over food—that our lives had become unmanageable.

2. Came to believe that a Power greater than ourselves could restore us to sanity.

3. Made a decision to turn our will and our lives over to the care of God as we understood Him.

4. Made a searching and fearless moral inventory of ourselves.

5. Admitted to God, to ourselves, and to another human being the exact nature of our wrongs.

6. Were entirely ready to have God remove all these defects of character.

7. Humbly asked Him to remove our shortcomings.

8. Made a list of all persons we had harmed, and became willing to make amends to them all.

9. Made direct amends to such people wherever possible, except when to do so would injure them or others.

10. Continued to take personal inventory and when we were wrong promptly admitted it.

11. Sought through prayer and meditation to improve our conscious contact with God as we understood Him, praying only for knowledge of His will for us and the power to carry that out.

12. Having had a spiritual awakening as the result of these steps, we tried to carry this message to others, and to practice these principles in all our affairs.

Permission to use the Twelve Steps and Twelve Traditions of Alcoholics Anonymous for adaptation granted by A.A. World Services, Inc.

THE TWELVE TRADITIONS OF ALCOHOLICS ANONYMOUS

1. Our common welfare should come first; personal recovery depends upon A.A. unity.

2. For our group purpose, there is but one ultimate authority - a loving God as He may express Himself in our group conscience. Our leaders are but trusted servants; they do not govern.

3. The only requirement for A.A. membership is a desire to stop drinking.

4. Each group should be autonomous, except in matters affecting other groups or A.A. as a whole.

5. Each group has but one primary purpose - to carry its message to the alcoholic who still suffers.

6. An A.A. group ought never endorse, finance, or lend the A.A. name to any related facility or outside enterprise, lest problems of money, property, and prestige divert us from our primary purpose.

7. Every A.A. group ought to be fully self-supporting, declining outside contributions.

8. Alcoholics Anonymous should remain ever non-professional, but our service centers may employ special workers.

9. A.A., as such, ought never be organized, but we may create service boards or committees directly responsible to those they serve.

10. Alcoholics Anonymous has no opinion on outside issues; hence the A.A. name ought never be drawn into public controversey.

11. Our public relations policy is based on attraction rather than promotion; we need always maintain personal anonymity at the level of press, radio, and films.

12. Anonymity is the spiritual foundation of all our traditions, ever reminding us to place principles before personalities.

The Twelve Steps and Twelve Traditions of Alcoholics Anonymous have been reprinted with the permission of Alcoholics Anonymous World Services Inc. ("AAWS").

"The whole world is ours, the whole of life, present and future,
scientific knowledge, artistic beauty, politics, eating and drinking,
sexual and romantic love, family life, friendship, justice, nature,
the technical world, philosophy in its true humility as the love of
wisdom, daring to ask the ultimate questions all belong to us."
                    --Paul Tillich, Pastor & Writer

 ll of these things are mine so long as I know and live in the self-truth of weakness, foolishness, reliance on my Higher Power, a God of my understanding, and move toward health. I will find wisdom and courage to view each day as an opportunity for happiness by focusing on the reality of today without the burdens of compulsive eating.

FOR TODAY: I revel in the new beginning of a New Year. I go forward in self-truth, discovered and to discover, recovered and to recover.

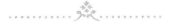

GIVING UP DESPERATION   JANUARY 2

"I have been a desperate person." --Anonymous

ecovery is a process. I accept the changes I will make. The tools and principals of the Twelve Step programs, patterned on A.A. - Steps, Traditions, Sponsorship, Meetings, and decisions about use of food plans and food -- can lead us to the answers that are right for us.

God, Keep me from being a desperate person.

FOR TODAY: I look to the New Year in joy. The need to survive and live well moves us on to better solutions.

"Take a rest; a field that has rested gives a beautiful crop."
-- Ovid, Philosopher

"Not eating for three days, staying up and then eating a super deluxe anything before crashing and sleeping for three days is exhausting. I can't do this anymore." --Anonymous

God, I am willing to take a rest from desperation. I know change is possible. With some knowledge of my messes and the challenges to come, I look into the New Year without lack or regret.

FOR TODAY: I am willing to use the tools and resources of a Twelve Step Recovery program to help me identify and deal with my desperation.

STRUGGLING   JANUARY 4

"The struggle for security is no picnic."
-Linus at Camp Snoopy, Charles Schulz, Cartoonist

If only I could achieve security and be free from fear... this is the great hope I jump at. I have followed a recommendation based on myths: first, that my weight or size or shape was to be altered by science; second, that my nameless fears were to be conquered and avoided at any cost; and third, that I should and would have immediate control over body size and weight forever. These myths are so popular in my culture.

FOR TODAY: I have other answers. The tools for living I discover in Twelve Step Recovery help me take care of myself. It is a good year. There will be more good things than things to fear in this bright New Year.

"He wants to lose 30 pounds for his date tonight." --Anonymous

ow I smile at 'magic think'. How I too have wanted love. How I want the instant perfect date. I have thought other people were having perfect dates. These ideas have taken the place of reality. I still want love. I know it comes from my heart. Belonging to myself first before I can love another is paramount. I know love comes from self-care first and having a self. My heart must belong to myself first, before I can love another.

FOR TODAY: I will tap into the one True Source of love and self-care, a loving God as I understand Him. I will laugh today. It will quiet my fears.

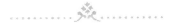

"I have been a fearful person." --Anonymous

ike an animal I have perked up my ears. I have lived in fear. Poison darts might strike me at any moment. Poison darts? Whose poison darts?

FOR TODAY: I know when danger comes from within and without. I have courage. I can take care of myself. I live in safety. I am compulsion free free today. I use my talents and develop new abilities and interests to be the basis of my identity - not my weight.

"My Mother took me to the doctor for my first diet pills."
                    --Anonymous

or many of us our Mothers took us to doctors for our first prescription diet pills. We weren't thinking for ourselves. We weren't thinking about the consequences, or the problem, or whether we had a problem and what it might be. The doctor wrote a prescription in a few minutes. I took the cure.

I know that my issues are complex. My path has been winding. Discussion about my issues and my path deserves more than a 15 minute consultation.

FOR TODAY: I make decisions. I give myself time to recover from faulty care. I ask all helpers to be God's agents.

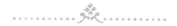

"I call a liquid protein and tangerine diet pretty weird. The liquid protein was made from horses hooves and looked like glue."
                    --Anonymous

he person who has done weird things with food - that person is in my heart. I don't beat myself up.

Today, when I hand over the garbage of my foolishness, I walk into a new moment. I am not alone.

FOR TODAY: I seek to understand and have compassion for the person I have been - that person is always in my heart.

"I wanted a free ticket. I was ready to fly."
                              --Anonymous

I have wanted - an edge - easy self-esteem - control - anticipated outcomes. I have wanted to be greater than - all the while having fear of being less than. I have wanted shelter from any storm – other people - banishment of fear – permanent ready-made security. Blast away. The only thing was, the diet pills and a chemical high have blasted away reality too.

I need to learn more about life, realistic expectations of myself and others, parameters for acceptable behavior, good times without harm, positive pleasures, and guides for living.

FOR TODAY: I am not the child with the hand in the candy jar seeking to pull all the candy out at once, losing most of it. Emptying my hands of some of my extreme wants makes life more manageable.

"All I ever wanted was to belong, to wear that hat of belonging."
                  --Anne Lamott, Writer

Belonging is so keen a want, especially at a young age. As we develop a self separate from our parents, we want to connect with peers. We want to do things that will make us acceptable and contributors so we will belong to society in the larger world. My fears have often driven me to behavior that grew out of my desires to belong. I have operated on misconceptions about what is required. When I am honest and authentic and develop a self, and am true to that self, I will find I belong.

FOR TODAY: I belong. I am God's creation, good and worthy, in community with others. I have been made to belong.

"Loneliness and the feeling of being unwanted is the most terrible poverty." --Mother Theresa, Nun

veryone feels lonely at times. Trying to be a different size or shape to escape the fear of feeling lonely is doomed to failure. I have made a misdirected attempt to escape this fact of life. I could not pour myself into a frozen form that had no feelings. I could not freeze my feelings. I am alive. I am flesh and blood. Feeling all our feelings is healthy -- a baby cries and laughs all in a minute.

FOR TODAY: I will sit with my feelings. I will not reach for an instant remedy. My Higher Power and members in the fellowship of Twelve Step Recovery help me identify my feelings and give me comfort. May I lean back on the everlasting arms of my HP in faith.

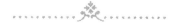

BEING A BEGGAR NO MORE   **JANUARY 12**

My best boyfriend said 'People only have as much power as you give them.' That's when I realized that I had been giving my power away to the wrong people. I gave away my power, until I almost lost myself due to dieting compulsively." --Anonymous

eeling unwanted makes us beggars. We expect from the other person. It gives all the power to others. I have started to care, really care, for myself. In recovery, I realize that others too are struggling to meet their own needs too. I want to care for myself.

FOR TODAY: I don't want to lose myself. I will not discount myself or give over my power for others to define me to fix me. I don't give my power to the wrong people. I have power to take care of myself.

"...with hideous conceit and low self-esteem.."
--Anne Lamott, Writer

Unsure of myself, outwardly conceited, arrogant, leaving home for the first time, entering the world, I have wanted transformation. I have wanted a way to break isolation of self. I have wanted to be popular, to win in the social competition. Taking diet substances or creating a chemical high from dieting, I have appeared six feet tall in the funhouse mirror. My head has expanded with flights of fantasy and conceit. Caution and humility has disappeared. It has been bizarre. Grandiosity and arrogance exist simultaneously with low self-esteem and fear. Taking chemical substances altered my perceptions of myself and the world.

FOR TODAY: I am not conceited nor filled with low self-esteem. I live in truth.

"I was in the drug store - they always say, did you find everything you were looking for? No, what aisle is the self esteem in, because the fake hair, nail polish, diet pills and Entemanns are not cutting it." --Vanessa Hollingshead, Comedienne

There is humor in some of my actions. What have I been looking for? Today I walk past the things I don't want or need in the drug store. I have no business cruising the aisles in zombiewalk, bored or directionless. My next step will become clear to me. If uncertain, I rest in the comfort of my Higher Power who will love me into the next step.

FOR TODAY: My road trip is planned in clarity, ahead of time, with plenty of rest. I put on my self-esteem and the shoes I like best.

"Perfectionism is a mean, frozen form of idealism while messes are the artists true friend." --Anne Lamott, Writer

The hard edges of perfectionism don't allow for kindness, mistakes, growth. Integrity is growth amidst mistakes and messes. Integrity allows me to move forward, accepting it all, and standing visible with strength.

FOR TODAY: I can be messy and still be a person with goals.

"Security is mostly a superstition. It does not exist in nature, nor do the children of men as a whole experience it. Avoiding danger is no safer in the long run than outright exposure. Life is either a daring adventure or nothing." --Helen Keller, Activist & Writer

I have often been afraid to venture out into life - like a cat that shakes its paw at the front door when it sees snow   I have been overly dependent, passive, and overly demanding of protection from others.   There is always the unexpected, beyond my control. It can catch me off guard, but I recover and respond the right way. I may not respond instantly or perfectly, but I know I will be able to respond. I accept the unexpected, knowing I can take care of myself. I strive for security at the soul level and at the habitat level - a habitat where I may safely live and prosper with family and loved ones.

FOR TODAY: Today I know there are rewards from venturing out. Life is an adventure. I turn the adventure into excitement. I don't need the cover of food, a substance, or false self. I take time.

"If you banish fear, nothing terribly bad can happen to you."
--Margaret Bourke-White, Photographer

I have been both afraid and fearless. On the one hand, I haven't been aware that I have been afraid. In fact, just the opposite. I have thought of myself as fearless, confident. But I have feared - people's looks, how I stacked up with others my age, whether I was as beautiful as, smart as, clever as. What would my future hold?

FOR TODAY: Whenever I have an attack of fear or self-loathing, or consider starting to compulsively eat, I check my inventory. What is happening? I identify my fears. In awareness, I discuss these matters with my Sponsor or trusted friends in Twelve Step Recovery.

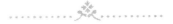

"I was not prepared for the difficulties of life. I had no idea how terrible youth would be for me. My innocence about it all is astonishing to me, perhaps even embarrassing. How could I have been so naïve?" --Anonymous

Nothing quite prepares us for growing up. Youth is about not knowing where to turn. It is about not knowing what next. It is about making decisions that turn out to be mistakes. A loving God is forgiving. A loving God wants us to grow and created us to grow in experience, light and wisdom.

FOR TODAY: Forgiveness. Cruelty is not in order. I can feel sadness about some aspects of growing up - then separate that feeling from regret and remorse.

"Remember that you own what happened to you. If your childhood was less than ideal, you may have been raised thinking that if you told the truth about what really went on in your family, a long bony white finger would emerge from a cloud and point at you, while a chilling voice thundered, 'We told you not to tell.'"
                    --Anne Lamott, Writer

Whether our Mothers were kind or were cruel, many had the aggressiveness and drive of a Joan Crawford in *'Mildred Pierce'*. They had an idea of what the perfect child should be and how they should act. Part of my recovery today is realizing my Mother's desperation and fear and forgiving her. Part of my recovery is separating from it and her.

FOR TODAY: I own my history and family history. The past is behind me. The future is not yet here. I live one day at a time in kindness and harmony and health. Great realities are open to me. I stop being desperate and deal with reality and food in a healthy way.

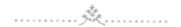

*"The hearts of children are delicate organs. A cruel beginning
in this world can twist them into curious shapes. The heart of
a hurt child can shrink so that, forever afterward, it is hard and
pitted as the seed of a peach. Or, again, the heart of such a child
may fester and swell until it is a misery to carry within the body,
easily chafed and hurt by the most ordinary things."*
                                        --Carson McCullers, Writer

I have heard children say things that are basically cruel in the guise of being powerful or knowledgable. They can have an arrogance not worthy of a child. Yet they are children. Often they have been frightened to death, scarred by scared desperate parents so they develop a punishing self. Today I recognize that thoughts and fears about weight and size begin at an early age. Fear and desperation pushes many of us to start punishing ourselves by taking our first diet remedies or using other methods for not eating, creating a chemical high to escape reality.

FOR TODAY: Seeing the hurt child in myself, or perhaps the hurting child or adolescent I became, hurting others with cruelty, helps me to put on the invisible, colorful, cloak of maturity. With the cloak of new beginnings, I am happy, kind to children, adults and myself alike, outgoing and beautiful.

How many years have I taken or used?

How many years have I used food compulsively? What methods have I used to diet compulsively? What was the progression of my illness? Was compulsive eating my affliction? Or compulsive dieting? Or both?

FOR TODAY: The road is long and winding. Today I move on to better solutions. I use real food in a regular and planned and aware way.

"If you set out to be liked, you would be prepared to compromise on anything, at any time, and you would achieve nothing."
                    --Margaret Thatcher, British Prime Minister

"When I lost my standards for everything else except weight loss any way possible, that was insanity. That was the extreme of isolation. It was loss of conscience." --Anonymous

FOR TODAY: Fellowship keeps me connected with a Source greater than myself. I pray and meditate. I talk to other members of Twelve Step Recovery groups at meetings and on the phone. Self-centered isolation is disappearing. I see the world is neither such a terrifying place requiring such extremes of feeling or action. There is greater kindness in the world than I imagined.

LEARNING ABOUT LOVE   JANUARY 23

"Where there is great love there are always miracles."
                    --Willa Cather, Writer

There is great love among recovering men and women in Twelve Step fellowship. Others in fellowship have experienced disappointment and punishment. There is great empathy, compassion and identification, and love for self and others. Together, patiently, I see compulsive behaviors disappear in others. I see my compulsive behaviors go.

FOR TODAY: I understand others in fellowship have experienced the punishment of compulsive eating too. It creates a bond of trust, looking for a common solution, personally right. I freely ask for help. I become free of conventional lies and biases. I become stronger in my decisions to speak up and act on what is healthy for me. I function better.

"It was a warm Fall day when my boyfriend and I walked to The Bagel on West 4th Street for breakfast. The walk was a romantic walk after waking up next to my lover. I was new to the City. I had made a big decision. I had moved to the City to live with him. I had decided also to stop taking diet pills. I had used them for 10 years. I told him I was stopping taking them. I also told him I was gaining weight. 'Isn't there something you can do?' he asked 'No,' I said. I knew the jig was up. I couldn't continue to take the diet pills. No matter what." --Anonymous

How do I know when enough is enough? Do I have to try every form my trigger foods are packaged under? Do I have to wait until I have tried everything on the drug store shelf or that the doctor has to offer to diet? Do I have to wait many years to see what next will come on the market? No.

FOR TODAY: I can gladly say - it was 'enough'. I make a realistic assessment, choosing what is healthy and good for me.

"The water is wide, I cannot cross o'er, and neither have I wings to fly. Give me a boat that shall carry two, and boat shall row my love and I." --O Waly, Waly, English or Scottish Folk Song

"Some girls had better bustlines in sundresses and smaller waists. My good legs wouldn't serve me until later. I was pretty demoralized and despondent. Angry at the way my life was written so far, I didn't have much faith when I started drug store diet remedies. I had been raised in a faith. I went to church with my family. However, my faith didn't seem to apply to something as real or as physical as my food or dieting behavior." --Anonymous

FOR TODAY: I have faith in the journey and the love that will help me. I cannot do it on my own. This is a "We" program of recovery.

"For something as physical as food and dieting, I had faith in self-will and science. Will power I was told was what I needed. Or science told me it wasn't a matter of will power. Science told me it could deliver good things. It could change my metabolism or my appetite or block food I digested." --Anonymous

We all believe in something. We put our faith in something. My new foundation is more in concert with teachings about self-regard for personhood. It has everything to do with inventory, respect for truth and the created world, and living on the basis of kindness toward myself and others. My faith in the created world is complimented by my knowledge from evolutionary biology showing each of us to have wonderful potentials and a unique combination of elements coming from our genes and nurture to be a survivor, coming from survivors, our ancestors in the river of time.

FOR TODAY: God wills my will to be, in concert with my conscience. I use my best lights to determine what is the best thing for me with use of real food in a regular, planned, aware way. I take actions to plan and eat my meals. I keep in contact with my Sponsor and listen to the experience, strength and wisdom of others in Twelve Step Recovery.

* * *

OBSERVING OURSELVES   JANUARY 27

"She ate penny candy and grazed for grapes." --Anonymous

We've been observed. "She ate penny candy and grazed for grapes." Some of us have used one kind of compulsive dieting method, some of us have used another. I too have observed roommates or friends or family members with their food behavior.

FOR TODAY: I have compassion and empathy. I identify. I relate.

"Going to the diet doctor was a well kept secret. The secret about my continued visits to the doctor for a refill kept me in shame. I was afraid to ask for a refill every month. If I lost or gained weight, or never achieved a real or imagined goal, I didn't discuss it. Usually we were both quiet while the prescription was written."
                                        --Anonymous

With the help of health-care professionals, non-professionals, and trusted friends in Twelve Step Recovery, I can discuss things in the open. Other people's hope, strength and experience shows me there is a body of experience on how to let go of diet substances, "diethead," and other methods I have tried. There is a better way, with the help of my Higher Power, to live life ethically, in health, joy, well-being, and usefulness.

FOR TODAY: I discuss things in the open.

"Watching pills disappear and worrying about dosages left and whether the doctor would give me a refill, created its own desperation. It wasn't like taking an antibiotic and the infection going away, indicating when to stop the drugs. If I lost weight, why couldn't I stop taking the diet pills?" --Anonymous

Fear has added onto fear. The problems caused by compulsive eating and dieting compound.

FOR TODAY: I list my fears. What products, substances, behaviors and methods and foods have I used compulsively. What foods have I eaten compulsively? Then I discuss them with my Sponsor and members in Twelve Step fellowship.

"How long I took diet pills worried me. They disappeared into my body daily. They worked or didn't work for 24 hours, then I took another one. Sometimes I didn't take a dose, to see what would happen. Those days were both a relief and dark. It was a relief not suffering the side effects of the diet pills. I could eat and sleep normally. I often binged. Worrying was dark. Days lapsed into months into years." --Anonymous

uman history is based on adaptation. We have the ability to learn - and to translate that learning into action. Experience - about planting a crop in the wrong place and not getting a yield - teaches what to do better the next time. Experience - about the water holes - teaches us where to go to get a good supply of running clean water. We build individual experience - we learn from that experience. We share our experience, strength and hope so others may learn.

God, Thank you for preserving my mind and giving me the will to want to live.

FOR TODAY: I want to live, free from harm. A new day dawns for me. I welcome it.

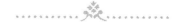

"You wore leotards; I wore leotards. You wore designer jeans; I wore designer jeans. You wore boots; I wore boots. The same brand. I went to a diet doctor. It amazed me when I found out you were going to the same diet doctor. I didn't know you had a problem with food because you were thin." --Anonymous

I learn in recovery that other men and women have problems with food. Others who share have used different methods to diet. Many have experienced side effects. Listening to others, I ask myself is my affliction overeating, or is it also about the masquerade, and the problems accompanying diet product use and chasing after the products to diet compulsively.

Many of us have been smitten with an insane urge to diet, overeat and or undereat.

God, Life is good. I have a chance to change my perspective. This chance is always available to me. I learn from others how to walk on brighter firmer paths. I will see the enchantment of life without chemical highs and lows of excess food or diet remedies or compulsive behavior. and I will share and participate actively, while thinking for myself. You will be my guide.

FOR TODAY: I choose carefully for myself what I wear and what I put in my mouth. I have the freedom to be myself. I create a style of living, rather than adopting one advertised that may not be right for me.

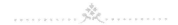

"To Thine Own Self Be True." --William Shakespeare, *Hamlet*

"I was a Wannabe. I wanted to be...anyone other than who I was. The pain was so great. The desire to escape led me to want to make myself invisible perhaps, to get rid of the me." --Anonymous

God, I am grateful for the Twelve Step program. The door is there when I knock and ask "Is it too late?" The answer is "No, C'mon in." The meeting is there for me. I am grateful for the teachings that all persons are uniquely themselves and worthy of regard.

FOR TODAY: Coming to the rooms of recovery with a willingness to be me, I am restored. I recover energy.

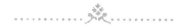

"If you are reading this, you are drawing on other people's experience, hope and strength." --Anonymous

I identify. I relate. I share my own experience, strength and hope with others because I care.

God, Thank you for preserving me and my life. I owe others more than I can return. Thank you for the recovery fellowship.

FOR TODAY: I am 'a part of' not 'apart from'. I am one among many.

"Fear is a question. What are you afraid of and why? Our fears are a treasure house of self knowledge if we explore them."
                    --Marilyn French, Writer

iet substances, appetite suppressants, central nervous system stimulants, diet herbs, boosters, blasters, blockers have operated to make me feel superior to my mere mortal friends. Underlying feelings of low self-esteem and fears were put aside. Getting along with others, operating in the real world, learning how to do a normal amount and take care of my body has been put aside as well. These real world skills I now know are important.

God, Take my desperation. Cover-up is unnecessary. I can do a normal amount. I can be equal to others, neither more than nor less than. I can walk on with the tools of the program, ever realistic and optimistic.

FOR TODAY: Pretending to be superior doesn't wash for me. When the desire to be superior comes up, I ask myself, "What is this about? What am I feeling shakey or defensive about?"

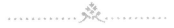

"Think wrongly, if you please, but in all cases think for yourself."
                    --Doris Lessing, Writer

ave I ever made mistakes? Through trial and error I have discovered some self-truth. In recovery I am encouraged to be guided by my Higher Power. Guided by my Higher Power I claim my self-truth.

FOR TODAY: I am grateful for the independence to live in self-truth. If not where I want to be, I am moving in a good direction.

"'When I get to be...[you insert the words], I'll get...[you insert the words].' Some of these magic-thinks might have been 'I'll get all the attention I want; I'll get whatever I want without asking for it; others will be mind-readers and will give me what I want; life will stop being hard; life will be easy...' I have 'gotten to be', [whatever, you name it], and the magic-think wishes didn't happen." --Anonymous

hese magic-think thoughts let me stay in the world of infantile omnipotence and fantasy. May I move beyond magic-think and resentments. I can set realizable goals and define how real needs can be met.

FOR TODAY: My resentments at the way life is lived are in transition. Seeing life as it is lived is an adventure. Setting realistic expectations is sanity. Developing and using my talents in satisfying ways brings me realizable rewards. I win.

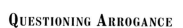

"I am the Queen of SIAM. I am I am." –Anonymous

randiosity is so invisible to ourselves. Characteristic of the spirit of youth, with its hopes, untried experiences, lack of real living experience, and false confidence, grandiosity puffs itself up. Sometimes it continues beyond youth. My grandiosity has driven me to feats of endeavor I could never attempt in maturity; it has hurt me when it set me up for a let down. My thoughts of self grandeur were not realistic and kept me apart from others.

Let me walk humbly with my God and my fellow human beings.

FOR TODAY: I smile with amusement at the grandiosity of my youth.

"When one person is diminished by prejudice, or by injustice, or by lack of opportunity, we are all diminished."
                                    --Kenneth O. Jones, Minister & Writer

 ruth is in our individual worth and dignity. Equality and justice extends to my treatment of myself. It is not just for others.

God, Let me remember, *"We gain strength because we are together in infinite variety and mesh our various and different qualities."*
--Kenneth O. Jones, Minister & Writer

FOR TODAY: I am not unjust to myself. There are acceptable practices for being in the world, safely, as part of civil behavior. I treat people with respect. I ask others to respect me.

TREATING MYSELF WITH RESPECT   **FEBRUARY 8**

"If you asked me to tap dance and recite from 'The Skin of Our Teeth', I'd try to please. Living on greens and throwing up like Elvira Madigan, Summer Stock had one of the most energized actresses before the Fall." --Anonymous

had to be better than other people, I thought. Love would come easily and perfectly to me, I thought. At the same time I thought I would have to work extra hard to have love come to me. None of it was true.

FOR TODAY: I look at my thoughts to see how far I have come in understanding.

When I idealize someone and think they are having more fun, or more romance, or more beauty or health, I remind myself, "I don't know that person. I don't know their health issues, their romance issues, their life issues, their past, or what their future will hold."

I don't know their strengths or weaknesses, or what they bring to the table in their work and relationships.

Idealizing is not living in real knowledge. It has no perspective. A dress, a curve of arm or back, a shape, may have its own elegance and attractiveness. However, it belongs to the holder, and to the great beauty in life. I won't use it to punish myself or to covet it.

I won't use any ideal to punish myself.

FOR TODAY: I won't use the ideal to put myself down. I see the good in me and others, in my relationships, my goals, my industry, my enthusiasms, and my work.

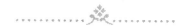

"*I thought there was an ideal man – young, preppy, no baggage, well-to-do, and eager to spend his money on me. When a date, a lawyer, suggested we split a bowl of soup and a sandwich at the Carnegie Deli, I flipped. I wanted my own. His previous girlfriend had been a petite iceskater. Here I was a thin hungry former diet pill user – and he was asking me to split a bowl of soup and a sandwich.*

In New York I visited MOMA – the Museum of Modern Art. There I saw the book of photos 'The Family of Man.' It influenced my thinking in seeing beyond my suburban small family of origin.

I also saw an exhibition on chairs. There was the fur-lined teacup chair and the angular Charles Eames chair. As I laughed and marveled at the silliness of the fur lined teacup chair, I asked myself 'what is this art exhibit saying?' All I could come up with was it was about seeing textures, contours, shapes, colors, design. There was no ideal chair. "--Anonymous

FOR TODAY: I see and revel in the textures, shapes, contours and colors of reality.

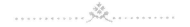

"My definitions change. Once I thought the girl across the street had it made. She worked at the deli – and was thinner than me - and had a sandwich named after her – the "Cindy Lou." It broke my heart I didn't have a sandwich named after me. She must have had love. I wanted a sandwich named after me. I had a mad crush on a dark haired Italian guy behind the counter. Maybe she had him. Never mind that I was working in a major publishing house in my dream job." --Anonymous

How I have wanted love. My ideas have often taken the place of the reality going on before me. How those ideas have driven my thinking and acting.

Love is not an isolated incident practiced with a certain person at a certain time of day. Love is in the world and in me and in other people when I become genuine and authentic and real.

FOR TODAY: My definitions change. What I am willing to see as good, desirable, nurturing, has a great deal to do with my willingness to receive love and to recognize it all around me.

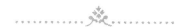

"I cannot afford to love but a few and be indifferent to the many."
--Anonymous

I have pinned my love on my small circle of family, or a few love objects. Then there has been heartache or death. I felt tragically heartbroken. My small world was shattered. All love was lost. What a resentment! Grief is real, and should be acknowledged. However, I often held onto resentment because of narrowmindedness. Self-centeredness deprived me of the fullness of love to be found in many people.

Great spiritual leaders, the great poets, the great leaders have loved the many and the individual. Jesus, Walt Whitman, Abraham Lincoln have each gone beyond the confines of their own time and place and family circle and personal tragedies to love.

FOR TODAY: I cannot afford to love but a few and be indifferent to the many.

Expressions of Love - Expressions of Tenderness

As Valentine's Day approaches I may be worried that I won't have my share. I may experience feelings of having less than, being lonely. If I "don't get" what is being sold as an expression of love, I may forget that there are all kinds of expressions of love, and I have received some wonderful expressions of love in my life over the years.

FOR TODAY: I count the special times and ways people have given to me. I count the special ways I am safe, cared for, given the space I need, the food, the shelter, the attention. Often it has come from unexpected places and in unexpected ways. People value and respect me. I am loved. I see it. I count the expressions of love.

"Amor and Psyche have been players on the field of love for ages -- apart from anyone's use of diet substances. Love and ideal love and our capacity for love with and without wisdom exist in the human psyche. Shakespeare wrote sonnets about it "

--Anonymous

As I learn more about love, I am more able to separate it from my ideas about use of diet substances and compulsive dieting. Sex addicts anonymous is a program to recover from sexual addiction. Some of us have had the affliction of romantic addiction. Romantic addiction means feeling you can't live without a person, will die if they leave you, will do anything to keep them, are distracted, totally powerless over thoughts of the romantic object. Romantic addiction has played into and fueled my use of diet substances and dieting compulsively. As I learn more about romantic addiction, I am able to separate it from my compulsive dieting affliction. I can see how my obsessions have played into one another.

God, This is the day set aside for the celebration of Romance. Whether my experience has been less than satisfying or satisfying so far in this area, let me keep my gifts in front of me.

FOR TODAY: I count knowledge and wisdom I have received as a great expression of love. Wisdom from my Higher Power and the fellowship helps me survive in health. I experience freedom and independence to develop my identity. I bring my attributes, ideas, humor, textures, contours and talents to others in the world for them to enjoy.

Admiring someone is natural

O ften my admiration immediately goes to envy and self-ruin. They have a figure I would die for. So starts the self-punishment and grueling behavior. A good day can be ruined in the blink of an eye.

FOR TODAY: I let go of reactive thoughts of envy.

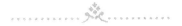

Compare & Despair

W hen I see people as opponents, rivals, competitors, winners, I start the comparison game. Don't even try to play that game, I tell myself. I don't need to give my power over to these thoughts.

FOR TODAY: What is this feeling? Let me recall that we are both beating hearts, breathing good oxygen, having the potential to grow, learn, and live in the sunshine of the spirit.

"A spiritual release comes when I can say 'Goodbye' to comparison. Letting others go on their journey and wishing them in lovingkindness 'God Be With You,' I release them to go on their journey. I have my journey and God is with me too."

--Anonymous

 etting go of comparison gives me release. It's no contest.

FOR TODAY: I will not see anyone as an opponent, rival, winner in relation to myself. It is unnecessary for me to assign people these roles. I give up these dramas. Today I keep the focus on myself, my life, my good attributes, building on identity, by living life as I go.

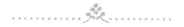

"I thought romance would come in a certain way. It would appear in a form I had imagined. It would meet expectations I had. When the romance or the person didn't meet my expectations, it was my expectations that let me down. The people were being themselves. Their purpose in life was not to meet my expectations or conform to my likes or dislikes." --Anonymous

ove comes in many forms, once we learn to recognize it. Because of my expectations of how love would come, I have been driven to diet compulsively. Sometimes we celebrate life. Sometimes we bump and kiss.

FOR TODAY: I have realistic expectations. I love the romantic feeling. I recognize it when it appears.

"She has composed, so long, a self with which to welcome him..."
                                    -Wallace Stevens, Poet

reparing a self to give to someone is an image archetype strong in our psyche. Wallace Stevens writes about it in the poem *"The World as Meditation"*, where Penelope is at home weaving waiting for Ulysses to return to her. The theme is repeated with the sleeping Princess waiting in the castle for her Prince to awaken her.

Preparation and waiting have been intricately involved with my use of diet substances and dieting compulsively. I thought that I was preparing myself to attract or attracting my suitors. Short-term weight loss may have been exciting. But patterns of self-punishment and tyranny were set in motion that I became powerless over.

FOR TODAY: I am worthy. I am relaxed in developing an art of living that I can bring to others.

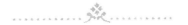

*"I am an actress. When the applause is over I go home by myself.
I compulsively eat or don't eat or take pills to feel the love.
It doesn't work."* --Anonymous

How often I have looked for approval from outside myself. Low self-esteem has driven me to constantly seek outside approval. Either I have been shy and silently sought approval. Or, I have been a super driver driving myself to great feats of work or service, hoping to prove to others that I was worth something. Liking myself is more important than momentary applause or praise. I realize I spend more time with myself than with anybody else. I live with myself 24/7.

FOR TODAY: I approve myself. Today I choose to travel first class with good company liking myself.

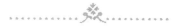

"Our school education ignores, in a thousand ways, the rules of healthy development."
        --Elizabeth Blackwell, 1st U.S. Doctor of Medicine

"Thirteen going on thirty. I put on stockings and bra and garter belt. All grown up. My school and my parents taught very little about the lifetime we are allowed to mature in health."
        --Anonymous

FOR TODAY: I dress for the day, appreciating my style and gifts. Being an individual in awareness of my unique response to life, is wonderful. I can't be all grown in a day.

"Keep us from any pessimism which may be induced by corruption, or by personal disappointment Keep us from defeatism and depression of spirit; for the promise is within the possibilities of our own experience: we can be changed."

--Kenneth O. Jones, Minister & Writer

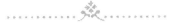

My first real adult disappointments were a big shock. We come from a culture that teaches only how to strive for happiness. Our first heartache may be our first real experience of disappointment. People aren't who we wished them to be. They didn't play the parts we had assigned them. We can think that we are the only ones disappointment has ever happened to. We might think there is something wrong with the feeling or with us. My pain of disappointment is intensely personal, no matter who else has had the same disappointment.

God, You are the Power of change within me, in times of sorrow and in good times, helping me move beyond disappointment. Let me be ever realistic but ever optimistic.

For Today: I identify feelings of disappointment as they happen. Let me stop. Collect. Grieve. Recover. Move on.

"When I decided who could win, I stacked the deck against myself. There are all kinds of winners." --Anonymous

Today I see there is a wider arena for success, or many arenas, in fact. Competitors - Winners - Losers. This is part of a losing mindset. It is a setup for resentments and anger.

For Today: I am a winner. I use my talents, abilities, industry, and enthusiasm today, and I am rewarded in real terms.

"If I was at a party and a woman spoke to a guy first, I saw her as a detractor. My reptile brain got so vicious. I was stunned and paralyzed with resentment." --Anonymous

I want what I want, when I want it, in the social arena. The "competitors - detractors - winners" are phantoms I create. They vanish as soon as I am willing to let them go, focus on my own abilities, and build identity by living life. This thinking about other people being better than me and me being in a contest has played into me taking diet substances and dieting compulsively.

God, I pray for clarity, to see myself as a real part of the picture. I exist. I have potential.

FOR TODAY: I see the world is a big wide wonderful world, with lots of arenas and possibilities for success, a moment to be well lived, and a future not yet here, with good things around the corner.

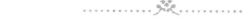

GOING IT ALONE   FEBRUARY 25

"I was told 'You're on your own' by my brother. It was sink or swim. Competing in adolescence and young adulthood sent me into superdrive. It was me against the world in a tyrannical competition." --Anonymous

Being on my own and needing people can be difficult. God, Help me acknowledge your providence and enlightenment. I don't have to go it alone. It's not me against the world. It never has been.

FOR TODAY: Because life is both a single adventure - we are alone and on our own with our individual talents and potentials and needs - and a cooperative venture - I use my individuality and live in interdependence.

"I must win all the time." --Anonymous

I want to win all the time. So do most people. The child who will not share, the child who gets upset at losing -- that is me. I don't have to be "the" star. I have my own bright lights. There are many stars. I am not invisible. I will contribute. Others also are not "stars," in the sense of having no trials, no flickers to their bright lights. The movie stars have their load of problems. I strive for health. I want you to have health also.

FOR TODAY: I honor and appreciate that person who wants to win all the time. I realize, however, that I am not omnipotent and cannot win all the time. Life cannot be lived without sharing and without having all kinds of players winning at all kinds of things. Superdrive will drive me to compulsively eat and or diet.

"We found, too, that we had been worshippers....Had we not variously worshipped people, sentiment, things, money and ourselves!" --*Alcoholics Anonymous*, Third Edition

Minnie Mouse, Olive Oil, Betty Boop, Barbie, Bratz Dolls, Anime. The first idols were amusing. Then the "wanabees" kicked in. Worshipping the "i-dollized body types" on the dolls, then later in the star magazines and on TV - instead of amusing or fulfilling me, left me empty and depleted. To be sexier than, prettier than, richer than... My real needs were filled by closeness to real people who focused on my need to build identity, my identity.

FOR TODAY: Friendship. Fellowship. Worship. We are together - in the same boat. I can ask, what does "worship" mean to me, and what is it appropriate to worship? Whether my Higher Power is a Higher Being or a Higher Power found within myself or the group, or some other understanding of God, I find satisfaction in worshipping a God of my understanding. I value spiritual progress.

"The voice of authority is not necessarily the voice of competence."
--Gerda Lerner, Women's Studies Writer

Many of our ideas about weight control and body image were the net result of lessons we and our parents took from the popular conture about how what we should look like and how we should deal with our bodies. We have been good students all our lives. We have learned lessons from parents and school. We have educated ourselves from the media. We have heard all the injunctions "you should do this; you should do that," especially about losing the pounds. We have thought there was an ideal size and everyone was cut from the same mold.

The child, the student in me thought whatever anyone said was probably true. Why else would they say it? Then I started thinking consciously for myself. I now evaluate what others say, to hold a gentle distance. Is it true? Is it kind? What can I learn from it. Is it life enhancing. Or, if there is nothing to learn from it, how can I quickly and easily discard what is irrelevant or just plain wrong.

FOR TODAY: I question. I reflect. I pray and meditate. I discern. From these actions I make my decisions.

"We're starting to see more and more anorexic eight- and nine-year-olds. It's a game we cannot win. Every time we agree to play another round and step out onto the court to try again, we've already lost. The only way to win is to stay off the court. No matter how much of our time is spent in pursuit of physical beauty, even to great success, the Mirror on the Wall will say, 'Snow White lives,' and this is in fact a lie -- Snow White is a fairy tale. Lies cannot nourish and protect you. Only freedom from fear, freedom from lies, can make us beautiful, and keep us safe. There is a line I try to live by, spoken at the end of each Vedanta service: And may the free make others free."

--Anne Lamott, Writer

I have tried many things: not eating, liquid fasts, appetite suppressants, central nervous system stimulants, diet boosters, diet blasters, diet blockers, diet bitter herbs, diet herbal teas, diet powders, diet liquids, diet pills, diuretics, purging, laxatives, punishing exercise, prescription drugs, over the counter drugs, compulsive exercise or combinations and variations of all of them.

I know that the desperation, the fear, and the self-punishment are the same no matter what compulsive dieting technique I am using. I need tools for living, including methods of being kinder to myself and others. I need to have a healthy relationship with food and eating regular meals. I need ways of being in the world safely.

God, Keep me from regret, worry and remorse over my past and allow me to be present in this bright new day. You are with me on my journey, in sorrow and fear, and in good times and growth. You lead me to greater mental and physical health.

FOR TODAY: I seek and find mental and physical health.

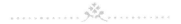

"Over the years I have taken everything on the market, including a few that were pulled from the market. It seems like every time a new savior is put on the market, in two years it is pulled from the market in a scandal and class action lawsuit. The company has made and taken the money and run. Hurt people are left. I noticed this but was powerless. The next "safe" diet substance or diet program advertised - I was first in line. What made me stop is another story." --Anonymous

What started out as an experiment may have become a lifestyle. A list of what we have tried, the years, the durations, may reveal that we have more of an affliction with dieting experimentation than we thought.

FOR TODAY: I look at my behaviors. I address my compulsie overeating.

STARTING TO DIET COMPULSIVELY   MARCH 3

"I have wanted to be the Goddess of Love. I have grabbed every food because I didn't want to miss out. I have grabbed every diet remedy. Girlfriends have divorced or stayed married. Children have been born healthy or not healthy. Men have left or stayed. I have been the Goddess of Love for a day, a week, a year, a few years. My ideas of triumph have changed." --Anonymous

Before I came into recovery, grabbing and conquering by every means may have been my method. Assumptions about triumph have not been a good basis for living. Accepting life as it is, living ethically, is a stronger basis for living than feelings about needing a triumph.

FOR TODAY: Satisfaction comes. During the course of the day I identify what gives me satisfaction and joy. In my inventory tonight I recall these satisfactions.

"I love the sweet talk of a man; I bought into it. When action didn't follow words, I had to recognize sweet talk for what it is. I loved that sweet talk of the food and diet program claims. Fools paradise. The purpose is to keep me in there." --Anonymous

 ood and diet claims, like alcohol for the alcoholic, have created problems for me. They have kept me in there while torturing me.

FOR TODAY: Sober health is my best friend and God-given.

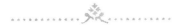

"I felt like a greyhound at the race track chasing the mechanical rabbit. The rabbit kept going round and round. There was no end. I couldn't stop." --Anonymous

I couldn't stop eating compulsively. Then taking diet substances to lose weight, then to maintain weight loss, then because I was afraid of regaining the weight, then because they stopped working, then because my body changed, then because they took one off the market for bad side effects and I had to start with another, then because I was afraid to stop, then because I couldn't stop, I see all the methods I have tried clearly now. Living in an ever-receding horizon of tomorrows isn't living well in today. I can stop compulsive chasing.

FOR TODAY: The only thing I have and the greatest thing I have is TODAY. I take on tasks to build and use my talents. I put positive joys in today. These are strong positive boundaries against the "when" mindset.

" I'm tired of living in the bottles, the packages, the bully parlors, and the toilets. Giving over my power has been demoralizing. Buying every diet claim has kept me poor. I have spent staggering amounts of money on diet claims." --Anonymous

I don't want to be a zombie, a pillhead, a diethead, or a dieter who will do anything. Yet I want answers for my compulsive eating. God gave me my own talents to be used today. Self-esteem begins with being honest. My Higher Power has given me a good life to live. I come into Twelve Step Recovery because I believe there is a Higher Power who will restore me to sanity. I can work out my todays beautifully together with others who share our common problem. We are powerless over fruitless compulsive behaviors. We need better solutions to problems of living.

FOR TODAY: I am made perfect and good. There is Wisdom in how I am put together, the Wisdom of the body, and centuries of selection to bring me here. I choose to place my trust in my Higher Power.

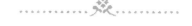

"I was swimming - side stroke - and was stiff from no movement. Slowly I felt my body loosen up. Slow growth. Swimming that day, in the Swim Club on the 25th floor of the World Trade Center Hotel -- I fully appreciated the slow growth. I was on Top of the World. I hadn't taken a diet pill or diet remedy in 25 years. That swimming pool in the sky is no longer there. It went down with the World Trade Center bombing." --Anonymous

I respect my own pace.

FOR TODAY: I respect my pace. I honor slow growth.

xcessive guilt, faulty assumptions about the world, untested self-image, perfectionism, wondering if I would do it right, has stopped me.

God, teach me that my regrets don't mean the end of the world. There are new opportunities for living life. I let the world meet my needs. I share with others.

FOR TODAY: I am consciously aware. I say "I want" and "I need." I am not afraid. I go forward. I want and I need affiliations, relationships, joys, livelihood.

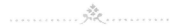

AVOIDING LIFE - LIVING LIFE   MARCH 9

"I thought life would be easy. What I wanted would fall into my lap. Parents and teachers sang songs of praise and love. Then when it wasn't that way – 'Stop the world, I want to get off.' Resistance. Rebellion. Defiance. I whined and thought – ' I need to be a student a little while longer. I need more education. I need to focus on my weight loss as my number one priority a little while longer. I need to stay in bed.' I went kicking and screaming to my first jobs. I was outraged at my first love breakup."
                    --Anonymous

 here are more satisfactions than kicking and screaming or avoiding life. Can I develop those talents seen by parents and teachers? Yes - by slow specific action. I gain satisfaction from self-generated effort and achieved competencies. Slowly they come.

FOR TODAY: Am I willing to have faith and belief? From a willingness to live life, I adapt, I learn, I discover. Thank you, Lord. With my talents and abilities, I live life. I discover more as I go. The ground meets my step.

"That Summer I turned 17. My first boyfriend came to the house. I got luggage for a high school graduation gift. The sounds of the radio turned into live concerts on green grass lawns. I started taking diet remedies. My Mother died. I started smoking cigarettes from the diet stimulants. I got accepted to go to college out of town. I cried." --Anonymous

I have focused on the pain of body image and comparison as one of my coping mechanisms for masquerating unnamable pains. A lot has been going on - as I prepared to leave home, started to live on my own, dealt with the difficulties of educating myself, working, being in a relationship, and assuming adult responsibilities.

Eating compulsively and dieting compulsively may have been a necessary distraction. It created a hope the pain would go away. It didn't work. It didn't get rid of the pain at all. The pain wasn't in my stomach.

FOR TODAY: My real needs are - the desire for opportunities, the desire for identity, strength, being in the world, safety, security, abundance, joy. I go about meeting my real needs today. I work at it. Life unfolds. The world meets my needs.

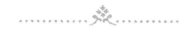

*"Beating myself up, then feeling guilty over eating, then doing extreme dieting, doesn't make me holy. It is not a cure. When I do my inventory and turn over the wreckage of the past, there is no cause for guilt. It doesn't change the fact – I wrecked the car on my way to the 7/11. Cars can be repaired." –*Anonymous

od, Let me separate the false regrets and guilt from the real. More of my regrets and my guilt are false and unreal than they are legitimate. I see my compulsive eating for what it is - a coping mechanism and an illness.

FOR TODAY: If I feel badly about anything, I will ask myself what is going on. I will "unbundle" the feelings. I will ask myself what, if anything, there is to feel guilty about. Maybe "feeling bad" is about other feelings – feeling sad, feeling disappointed, grief, feeling about someone's elses troubles or pain. I will look clearly at my feelings. I can sit still safely with them without trying to repair or get rid of the feelings.

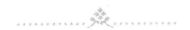

"Starving myself was once a habit. Restricting what I ate to not eating at all gave me a chemical high. The euphoria was just like a drug. I became addicted to being hungry. You reach a stage in life and maturity where you realize you can get a much deeper gratification from accomplishing things in the real world than from starving yourself." --Kate Taylor, Writer

I have spiralled out of control with restricting what I ate. Any pleasure from it is gone. I was a prisoner held captive from a behavior pattern that didn't work. I have a better answer now with healthy use of real food. My life is no longer unmanageable with a lifestyle dieting compulsively, or an identity based on this behavior. Today, I take my food with me. I have it prepared. I eat it. It is my trusty friend. Near me, I don't have to think about it - or stave off hunger when it is time to eat a meal. I have my food.

FOR TODAY: The frenzy is replaced with a regular committed plan for eating.

APPEARING TO LOOK GOOD   MARCH 13

""I wish I was like you. You're so beautiful with your boots, your make-up. I've gained 4 pounds and I have to go on stage,' my best friend said. 'Even if you were 4 pounds less, it's your insides that are making you still feel unattractive. It's the thinking,' I replied."
--Anonymous

I want to travel first class with my thinking and attitudes. They say "Don't compare your insides with their outsides," in Twelve Step Recovery. They mean someone may look good, but feel badly. Letting go of "stinking thinking" is part of my recovery.

FOR TODAY: Looking good doesn't wash if I don't like my behaviors and attitudes. I want to practice kindness, love and tolerance, and usefulness.

"Recovery is like a big old house... The anorexic or bulimic is always going to live there... I prefer to think of it this way. She used to rule the house in a kind of tyranny... Now she still gets to live there." --Sheila Reindl, Writer

ompulsive dieting has given me a sense of control, rigid restriction, like an aescetic who could deprive herself, as though punishment itself were the goal. The behavior has given me a sense of doing something about uncomfortable feelings I could not deal with.

Today I pray in gratitude for continued safety and preservation. It is new thinking not to tyrannize myself.

FOR TODAY: Finding a place where I am safe and respected for me, where I can share some of my feelings and learn the tools for living, is a wonderful gift from my Higher Power and the Twelve Step Recovery fellowship.

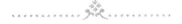

"My culture imposes restrictions as part of being female. Restrictions of clothing -movement - place. It has gotten better. Still, I thought my job was to restrict and prohibit myself and others. I related dieting compulsively to being feminine. I thought being cruel and restricting myself and others was a woman's job."
                                    --Anonymous

oday, my appreciation of my femininity doesn't require dieting compulsively.

FOR TODAY: I use wise-mind in deciding my behavior.

"You can't be in a relationship alone. When I have been in good, positive life-affirming relationship with someone, they are in the relationship. I am not alone. God is the divine Third in the relationship too." --Anonymous

 llowing others in means letting them love me. It has nothing to do with restricting my size or shape or weight.

FOR TODAY: Allowing others in is a joy I let happen.

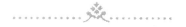

rothers and fathers, boyfriends and husbands, friends and loved ones have been powerless over our compulsive eating and dieting. They have seen the destructive results on character, behavior, and health.

FOR TODAY: The messages to restrict, so much a part of my culture - 'you must do this' - won't distract me from using my wise-mind. I know what is healthy for mind, body and spirit. My Higher Power helps me live today with courage in recovery.

"One pill makes you small... Go ask Alice."
   --Grace Slick, Songwriter; Jefferson Airplane, Rock Band

I have tried being invisible, quiet, a shy wallflower. Shrinking, perhaps, would let me avoid conflict. Shrinking, along with people pleasing and de-selfing, might make me totally fit in and be acceptable. And liked by everyone! Animals shrink or crouch to appear small or weak to avoid conflict with a stronger, superior, or bullier foe. Shrinking down also represents a body position, if we think we have done something wrong. Trying to be be invisible is a defense mechanism.

Alice in Wonderland took a pill to shrink in *Through the Looking Glass*. When she took another pill, she was made large and unwieldy breaking out of the house. She couldn't win with those pills.

I have tried being invisible and have found it wanting. Trying to hide only denies my reality and my truth. I exist. I face the world in integrity.

FOR TODAY: I learn answers here and in Twelve Step Recovery for how to deal with my fears and be safe in the world. I do not need to try to be invisible. I greet each new day in confidence.

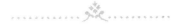

"'What are you on?' he said." --Anonymous

We may try to be invisible. But we aren't invisible. Loved ones, employers, co-workers see our behavior.

FOR TODAY: My behavior is knowable, predictable. They know me at work. I show up as a regular person for my responsibilities.

"At my youngest and thinnest, I thought I was not adequate to the job of living." –Anonymous

oes she have big feet - small feet? Big breasts - small breasts? Big hips - small hips? Big butt - small butt? Bigger than mine? Smaller than mine? What a waste of time. I'm never going to be that person. Body sizing is pretty shallow -- though interesting, because human beings are interesting, and we live in a visual physical world.

I need to stay away from sizing people up – including sizing myself up. My assessments are colored by the glasses I am wearing. Wearing the "what's wrong with this picture" glasses, I have blamed and criticized myself and others. Sizing up with these "what's wrong with this picture" glasses allowed me to justify isolating, eating compulsively and then dieting compulsively.

Why not change the glasses to "what's right with this picture?" Why not work with what I've got?

FOR TODAY: Sizing myself up is something I leave to my Higher Power. In daily inventory, I include "what's right with this picture" in my inventory of my day's activities. I include "what's right with me" in my thinking today.

"Tensions may be relieved and hearts attuned to be receptive to healing, forgiveness, grace, and love."
--Kenneth O. Jones, Minister & Writer

Once I started sharing my secrets about my illness with compulsive overeating and dieting compulsively, so much tension was relieved. I was not alone with my secrets. I became open to not holding in.

I receive the comfort of knowing I have made the best decisions I could at the time.

Many times I have wanted to change my physical outsides so I could get close to people. I sought a way out of loneliness. In Twelve Step Recovery I find the gift of bonding and affiliation.

The Ninth Step in Twelve Step Recovery says: *"Made direct amends to such people wherever possible, except when to do so would injure them or others."* Step Nine also applies to my sharing. It reminds me not to harm myself or others in what I say, or in the time and place where I say it. I choose the right place and time for sharing. I choose health-care professionals, non-professionals, counselors, trusted friends in fellowship, and my Sponsor to share with.

FOR TODAY: Being alone with my secrets is gone. I am in the present now. I move on and share with others about other things about me and live, all in the right time and place.

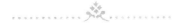

"Herbs. Supplements. That's what the diet programs call them. They are marketed to suppress appetite, stimulate metabolism or block digestion." --Anonymous

D ressing up diet remedies with pretty names, euphemisms, doesn't cover up the fact that they are being sold as ways to suppress appetite, stimulate metabolism, block digestion, promote elimination, or change body composition. My obsession jumps at the pretty sounding names. Pretty packages with crinkly sounds and colorful wrappers dress up my trigger foods.

It requires me to be vigilent not to jump. The packages and the advertisements promise novelty. If I am bored, perhaps the dressed up substances or trigger foods might be a way to quell my boredom, a distraction. My Higher Power has given me talents and time to use with purpose and direction.

God, Let me focus on basic good realities of the day ahead - getting up, washed, being clean, dressing with clothes I enjoy, clicking into how I will smile and contribute today, thinking about and planning my food for the day, taking care of other responsibilities for the day, one step at a time.

Extra time provides me an opportunity to meditate, or to put on my "thinking cap." I decide what project I would like to focus on. What project would give me satisfaction by putting some time into it today? I need never be bored if I put my "thinking cap" on to guide myself away from boredom, toward meaningful and satisfying activites, today. I don't need to go near the dressed up diet products.

FOR TODAY: I put effort into my recovery. I plan satisfying activities and efforts to bring me satisfactions for the day. Putting joy into my enthusiasms and projects today, plays into building my identity, achievements, pleasures, and next steps for tomorrow.

"I have tried diet bully parlors, the tyranny of outside regulation from diet club counselors for my eating." --Anonymous

ullying is bullying, no matter who it comes from - myself or others. Doing what is right for myself, and making the effort, is different from bullying. With effort I develop and use my special abilities, gifts and talents in a creative way. With bullying or abuse, people are criticized for something about them, or they are asked to go beyond their limitations unnaturally, or they are taunted or coerced.

I observe the environment around me. I observe, just observe, how, when, and where there is bullying. Coercion is another form of bullying. Does it come from the media? From others? In my workplace? In my home? From me? Recognition goes a long way to clearing my head of any bullying or coercion that is going on - by whomever.

FOR TODAY: I observe. I recognize bullying, abuse, or coercion. I separate right behavior for me - from any bullying, abuse or coercion messages going on around me. Tyranny leaves. I focus on liking my behaviors - my eating and behaviors toward others.

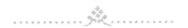

"Coming to Twelve Step meetings, I have learned other people have felt alienated and isolated too. I tried to change my size, shape, contours and weight to avoid these feelings." --Anonymous

All of life for humans is a process of becoming an individual, building identity. We are all different - especially when we develop our individual talents to make our individual contributions. We are normal and different from other people at the same time. I won't torment myself by taking diet substances or using other methods to diet compulsively to be "normal," to combat feelings of alienation, isolation, and differentness.

FOR TODAY: Discomfort tells me something about my differences from other people. I accept these differences and don't judge them as bad. I don't need to get rid of differences.

"I don't know -- they are making me feel kinda whacky."
--Anonymous

 My behavior had me monitoring myself every minute. I have been living on the edge.

We live less on the edge, more normally by having food and food times safely planned. It is easier to recognize the dinner bell as hunger. There is more time for living. We are safe. There is another meal coming. I believe I can live in physical and mental and spiritual health without overeating and dieting compulsively

FOR TODAY: Less self-absorbed now that I am safe, I focus on jobs, enthusiasms, my desires and specific actions to achieve in attainable ways. I focus on satisfactions, loved ones, small acts of caring, art, both making it and appreciating it, and the colors and sensations of the day.

"You're houseclearning at 4 a.m.?" he said." --Anonymous

hemical highs made behavior unpredictable. It kept us apart. Others could not understand what we were doing or why we were doing it. We were not operating on a level playing field with others in health or sanity.

FOR TODAY: It is important to me to be in the same world with others, not apart from them.

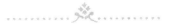

"'How good can that stuff be for you?' he said." --Anonymous

oved ones may have tried to talk to us about our behaviors. They may have known what we were using or not known. They may have suspected, but feared saying anything. They may have watched the diet and binge cycles, the yo-yo weight loss, and the frustration. Especially if aggressiveness, self-tyranny, tyranny of others, or dogmatism, characterized our behavior, what could they expect?

FOR TODAY: I open communication with myself, God, and another human being. It is more satisfying than keeping myself apart. I allow others in.

"Establishing a healthy relationship with food was not my goal."
--Anonymous

The joy of living my days in peaceful relation to food is a powerful goal today. It may be morningtime or nighttime as I read this meditation. Either way, I am in a good place. I am meditating on my behaviors, establishing goals and believing. I believe I can obtain emotional and physical stability. I believe in spiritual progress. These are good things.

FOR TODAY: Being able to give up the useless is growth. I claim new energy.

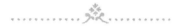

"If we had no winter, the spring would not be so pleasant."
--Anna Bradstreet, Writer

Moods change. Dark moods. Ebullient moods. Terrifying moods. Clear days. We have had many moods. In recovery we will have many moods. Moods come with living.

Moods are to be navigated. They can be navigated without dieting compulsively. I have weathered many storms. There is shelter in fellowship with the comfort from others. I gain wisdom from their stories of passing through dark times.

FOR TODAY: I am sensitive to my moods. Aware. They may change quite a few times during the course of today. I am ready - because it is natural.

"The new women in politics seem to be saying that we already know how to lose, thank you very much. Now we want to learn how to live." --Gloria Steinem, Feminist Writer

 e are each uniquely ourselves. Our experience is our own. We can recall what we have tried. Today, I must live. Today I must live with my whole heart. Meditating, gives me a perspective on my life.

FOR TODAY: Living and practicing life-affirming behavior is the answer.

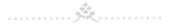

"No man is an island, entire of itself; every man is a piece of the continent, a part of the main... I am involved in the whole of mankind." --John Donne, English Poet

y personal experience could fill a book. It is valuable.

God, Life is given to me. Teach me to use things in their goodness, to see their goodness and their purpose.

FOR TODAY: I have an instinct to find my freedom in choosing good things.

"What happened to make me stop is a jumble of events culminating in a crisis. I had such a big head, filled with such grandiosity, and willful wishes. Nothing was good enough for me. I was poisonous. I was knocked silly by great expectations for perfect romance and easy living, and overstriving. The more I put it together, the more I knew how sick I had made myself. " –Anonymous

The wake-up call for each of us has been different. Our problems with food and compulsive dieting didn't develop overnight. Our recovery won't happen overnight.

God, I will remember "Footsteps". You have carried me in troubled times when I didn't see You. You are with me.

FOR TODAY: One day at a time, being comfortable with myself is a rewarding challenge. I love it. As painful as it is sometimes to recognize my negativity and faulty thinking, I open my eyes to the wonderful things in front of me in life. I heal. I enjoy life. I will never forget my wake-up call.

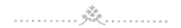

"Why all this insistence that every A.A. must hit bottom first? The answer is that few people will sincerely try to practice the A.A. program unless they have hit bottom. For practicing the remaining eleven Steps means the adoption of attitudes and actions that almost no alcoholic who is still drinking can dream of taking."
  --*The Twelve Steps & Twelve Traditions*, Alcoholics Anonymous

The voices of alarm are the voices that tell me to overstrive, compulsively overeat and compulsively diet. I have come into Twelve Step Recovery. I have started to make spiritual progress. I have made a decision to turn my will and my life over to the care of God as I understand Him. I have started to give up diets of my own willful making. I have started to choose a firmer brighter path to deal with food and life. I take direction in humility. Taking direction is a first for me. I am learning how to get along. I am willing to accept my problem is not compulsive overeating or compulsive dieting alone. I am bringing humility with me everywhere.

FOR TODAY: I know reality. I no longer live in the fantasy "just lose weight and everything will be alright." Life and living issues are in front of me to be engaged with happiness and excitement.

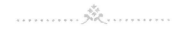

"Many a humble soul will be amazed to find that the seed it sowed in weakness, in the dust of daily life, has blossomed into immortal flowers under the eye of the Lord." --Harriet Beecher Stowe, Writer

Many of us were dumbfounded and scared when we walked into our first Twelve Step meeting. We were beat. How could this be happening to us? We had thought we were so smart. We would use science and willpower to win at the game of weight loss. Just losing weight, we would win at the game of life.

We were learning we did not have the control over food we thought we had. How could this new awareness change things?

Lord, Make Thy presence felt in my life. My life has been filled with a sense of inadequacy. I am not inadequate. I sow new seeds.

FOR TODAY: I thank my Higher Power I am alive and of sound mind. I am alive to the great possibilities in living. Each moment is precious.

"An eating disorder is one kind of translation, an action that 'acts out what the soul is feeling.... Your body is neutral and innocent, and it tells the truth. So instead of fighting it, pay attention to what it is trying to tell you.." --Aimee Lui, Writer

When I was younger, I didn't understand my body. My mind was the boss. Gradually I have learned that my body has a mind. I have to mind it. I am still learning, still listening. Learning respect.

FOR TODAY: I am willing to learn. My desire to control is not the boss.

"Hope is the power of being cheerful in circumstances that we know to be desperate." --Anne Lamott, Writer

ven though my behavior with food has been desperate, I have continued in the hope that something better would appear -- more courage to deal with my compulsion, greater honesty, greater courage to shift away from the behavior and the thinking. Hope is God-given. I have always had hope.

At the bottom of my despair - I have had hope. I have found faith. Hope is at the bottom of the Pandora's Box. When scary things fly out of the Pandora's Box and I look at them, there at the bottom is my hope. My faith is my willingness to continue in knowledge and wisdom.

FOR TODAY: I live in hope. Being cheerful, in the face of my tragedies and disappointments, accepting it all without judgment or blame, I see life as something marvelous.

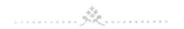

"With her fog, her amphetamine, and her pearls... "
--Bob Dylan, Singer-Songwriter

We have been observed. The people in our lives have watched us. Sometimes they said nothing. Sometimes they conspired and bought into it. They didn't know the problems it would cause us. Sometimes they abandoned us. Sometimes they left us to the winds of fortune, whatever they might be. I am not a freak. I take responsibility for self-care today. I am not blowing in the wind, a rolling stone, stoned, or part of the in-crowd or party with the soft or hard, street or prescription drugs. I am not high on diet substances or dieting. I am not in isolation either, stuck in my diethead. I find and take comfort in spiritual progress made with the help of my Higher Power and the Twelve Step fellowships.

God, I have gratitude to You, my Higher Power, for my survival.

FOR TODAY: I act in self-care. I practice neither absurd abandon nor just-as-capricious control. I am sane and sober. I am joyous in non-harmful ways. My personality comes through sublimely, because I am more than weight, and others who love me have always known this.

"The impulse is not the enemy. This mistaken notion is part of the myth that surrounds eating disorders. Like all self-destructive impulses, urges to restrict, overeat, or purge are distress signals – warnings that the body is under attack and in danger of overloading." --Aimee Lui, Writer

iet and binge cycles have been punishing. Suffering disappointment, considering myself a failure, I set myself up. These routines lowered self-esteem. I tried to self-medicate. I tried to control. I failed. The dieting was punishing. The binging was punishing.

God, I remember the word "spiritual" when I think about letting go of punishing behavior and low self-regard.

FOR TODAY: I can say - "Goodbye" - God Be With You - and let go of punishing behaviors. A spiritual release comes when I can say "Goodbye". They can take a hike over the horizon.

"Dancing to the tune of other people's likes or dislikes, a message from tv, radio or magazine, made me a beggar, a pauper, and a puppet. I had boyfriends who I gave all the power to. What did he think of this? What was he looking at when he tooked at me? Were the eyes critical or loving? How long could I keep his eyes loving? How long could I keep him?" --Anonymous

It is hard to survive in these lopsided arrangements. When I give all my power to someone else, it is hard to last. Sooner or later something has to give.

FOR TODAY: I recognize the performance stress I have put on myself, by performing to real or imagined expectations. I am a valuable, capable, albeit limited, flesh and blood human being. My Higher Power, who I conceive of as Great Mystery partly known and known about, has put me on the face of the Earth to struggle, adapt, discover, learn, survive, thrive. Helpers from parents on keep me in their loving eyes and give me help.

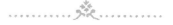

"Like the alcoholic who has been in an accident or a bad scrape, I got a startling wake-up call. I swore off. I found a Twelve Step meeting. I was one sick puppy. The safe haven of the rooms found me, startled, awakened - impoverished emotionally, spiritually, physically." --Anonymous

Facing danger means looking at it all - eating compulsively over many years, compulsive overeating, using many different diet methods. I know the whole life history.

FOR TODAY: I vividly recall my whole life history. I keep my memory green. I have been in a few scrapes – and I have survived them. Today is a new day.

WHAT HAPPENED TO MAKE ME STOP

"We need to make messes in order to find out who we are and why we are here." --Anne Lamott, Writer

Perfectionism and struggle to achieve a certain weight or shape has led me down a long messy road, strewn with pill bottles, diet substances, and artificial foods. The messes I made have given me first-hand knowledge. That knowledge is now part of my recovery.

FOR TODAY: Knowledge is part of my recovery. I am an artist of my life, using all of it to create my life.

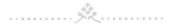

"She takes just like a woman....But she breaks just like a little girl." --Bob Dylan, Singer-Songwriter

It was a relief in some ways, hitting bottom. Hitting bottom has been uniquely my own experience, uniquely personal. Whatever it has been, it has given each of us the empirical evidence. Yes. I am a fragile flesh and blood human being. I can break.

FOR TODAY: I remember - I can break. There is happiness in not driving myself beyond my limits. I get well. I am not willing to kill myself to lose weight. I am going to be ok, more than ok. I am going to have well-being.

"What will happen when I stop?" --Anonymous

eing afraid to ask, and being afraid to express the question to another human being, comes from fear and pride. Complex questions and worries, mixed with pride, make for a bubbly brew. I won't sit in my own stew. It is esteemable to recognize this pride and communicate honestly and openly with another trusted human being.

FOR TODAY: Vagueness is not my friend. If the fog of pride is covering my eyes, I pray to have it lifted. My Higher Power helps me look squarely at what is bothering me and talk to another trusted human being about it. Otherwise, I am in the soup. I stew.

"Too much social pressure, holiday times, a new love interest, family tension, performance anxiety, and stress -- all of these could trigger the urge. The urge to use a diet substance, to purge, binge or starve, led to various types of mental and physical illness. Let's not tell our sad stories." --Anonymous

ne way to curb the urge is to observe it carefully and respect the message it is sending. In humility, in self-care, we keep the dangers of going out again in front of us.

FOR TODAY: I am adequate. I do what is given to me to do today. I keep my eyes on my own plate. I do not have to compete or overstrive to be fulfilled. The world is abundant enough for me. The problems can be handled without overeating or dieting compulsively. My health becomes better.

"My doctor tried to get me to have my stomach stapled. I told him that would be like cutting off an alcoholics leg so they couldn't walk to the bar for a drink. I knew no matter how small they made my stomach it wouldn't stop me from over filling it. Working the steps. Turning my life over to my HP and letting go of the anger and resentments I've been carrying around my whole life has started to actually stop that nagging voice that tells me it will take a lot more food than I see here to make me feel better. I'm not so anxious. I can enjoy meal times most days and can enjoy eating with my family again." --Anonymous

I remind myself daily - I am a recovering diethead. Anything that is suggested to me regarding diets or losing weight I might jump at. It took a lot for me to come into Twelve Step Recovery. This is where I belong. This is the life-affirming and health-giving answer. Today, clarity, self-knowledge, and an unwillingness to respond to alarming voices permits me to live the life God has given me and has preserved in joy.

I have an opportunity, one day at a time, to have a daily reprieve from the physical abuse and the negative thinking that accompanied my behaviors. I can continue to make spiritual progress by seeking daily to keep in conscious contact with my Higher Power through prayer and meditation. I have a chance to give up old assumptions about weight loss, about the world, and about my part.

FOR TODAY: I claim clarity and use my own wise-mind and my own voice.

"When I told the practitioner about the heart palpitations I was having from the diet powder, he said he could give me tranquilizers to stop that. It was at that point I decided not to compound my problem and risk death." --Anonymous

I have been spared much tragedy because I have used the intelligence God gave me. Sometimes my back has been up against the wall to learn. My Higher Power has given me that wall. In a thousand ways I have been spared. Others in recovery have forged the path. Although there is underbrush, and there are new obstacles and temptations to evaluate - I can see the path, sometimes ever so faintly - even when faulty information would try to point me in the wrong direction.

"God, We have been spared by Thy providential care the ten thousand dangers which could beset us." --Kenneth O. Jones, Minister & Writer

FOR TODAY: I value the life that has been given to me. I value the clear path I see. My lessons are hard won. I value my own intelligence – I will use it today and everyday.

RECOVERING NOT RECOVERED   APRIL 16

"It's hard to fight an enemy who has outposts in your head."
                    --Sally Kempton, Writer

The enemy that has outposts in my head - and would sabotage my recovery says - 'This way. Losing weight any way possible is your goal. This way to your goal...' They are banshees, space monkeys. They lurk around drug store diet product shelves.

FOR TODAY: I don't hang out with the drug store banshees and space monkeys, to act out with taking a diet product or eat compulsively and then diet. I am in a better position to work through my feelings, problem solve, and move toward constructive goals.

WHAT HAPPENED TO MAKE ME STOP

"Mistakes are part of the dues one pays for a full life."
                    --Sophia Loren, Actress

egrets can lead us toward a greater acceptance of life, as it is given to each of us. To regret deeply is to live anew. In the A.A. Twelve Steps and Twelve Traditions, it says, we did not understand how our sons could be killed in the war, or how some of us could be given healthy children and some none at all, or how our deepest disappointments could be given to us.

Thomas Merton, a Jesuit Monk, writes *"We are each completed by another. Our successes are not our own"*

By learning humility, we can see ourselves as a part of humanity. We can understand and take our part. We gain a greater understanding about the infinite variety in people and what makes us unique, and worthy of self-respect in all regards. Respecting our fragility is a good beginning toward respecting other things about our natures and abilities.

God, Make Thy presence felt in my life. Help me respect my part.

FOR TODAY: I regret. Yet, I wait to see what is around the corner. I can't see around the corner til I get there. I have already received some of my deepest desires. I respect my part in life.

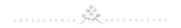

"Since I have been abstinent, I am healing from my compulsions to grab, use, buy into media messages or advertisements."
--Anonymous

Seeing "with my own eyes" takes precedence over media messages telling me what to believe or how to intepret the facts. I use my own mind, wise-mind with help from my Higher Power. Living my own life in health is always in front of me. I don't take in the alarming voices advertising weight loss products and methods. I don't buy into the packaging of the food.

FOR TODAY: I am aware, with a clear distance from alarming weight loss media messages.

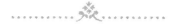

"People think that when something goes 'wrong,' it's their fault. If only they had done something differently. But sometimes things go wrong to teach you what is right." --Alice Walker, Writer

I thought it was my fault compulsive eating and compulsive dieting failed. It wasn't my fault. Learning in adversity was not fun. Being truthful about what went wrong is liberating.

God, My awareness of You in my life affects my decisions. I am aware of a new dimension for life-affirming, ethical, moral decision-making and action. and help available from trusted others. I am aware of compassion and kindness toward myself and others. With your guidance, I live honestly and conservatively. I don't take radical harmful actions to change my body. I am willing to live without fear.

FOR TODAY: I make the best decisions I can.

Why is it that there are some people who can drink alcohol and not become alcoholic? Why is it that diethead, compulsive overeating and then compulsive dieting, can alter thinking for some of us or become a consuming lifestyle? I am the only one who can decide if my life has become unmanageable. I know personally the thinking and behaviors. My decision is to stop being driven and to let my Higher Power and trusted others help.

FOR TODAY: Keeping the focus on myself, I use wise-mind to stay out of the road. Just like I don't get hit by a car, I stay out of the way of other people's opinions or judgments about what I should do. I avoid answers that are neither life-affirming nor moral or right for me. I don't impose my answers on others.

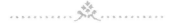

"Slow down. You're movin too fast."
> --Paul Simon & Art Garfunkle, Singer-Songwriters

Tag along behaviors: smoking, nervousness, sleeplessness, not eating at regular times, rushing, working too hard, isolating from family and friends, becoming secretive, becoming sexually compulsive, tyranny of children and spouse, attempted control of other people's food, aggression, a chemically altered mind, came along with compulsive overeating and compulsive dieting.

FOR TODAY: I can be still. Getting sober and clean opens a whole new world of relationships and behaviors. In Twelve Step recovery I can begin to question some of the abusive behaviors I have practiced.

"Sometimes it takes years to really grasp what has happened to your life." --Wilma Rudolpf, Olympic Gold Medal Runner

Seeing the healing may take a long time in a gradual awakening and awareness. The harmful patterns may have become so habitual they may beem normal. Seeing the depth and breadth of change when it does come may take many years to grasp.

At first we recognize "what happened," the toll on our physical and mental health, our interests, our relationships, our moral priorities. Then we see the "challenge ahead." Then we start "living in recovery", and "working a program of recovery," one day at a time. Living without requires new lessons in living. Others have forged the path. They are willing to share with us.

For Today: I may not be able to grasp yet how to recover. I trust I can learn new ways. Where there were walls, there are now windows and doors.

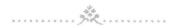

"The next few years were about healing....I was on the road to recovery, and though I had put all the weight back on, it finally occurred to me that when I'd lost the weight, I had lost myself. That conforming to a standard that was not developed with me in mind would be more counterproductive than good. I started to own my body, and I felt stronger and healthier than ever."
--Camryn Manheim, Actress

I t startled some of us how dieting compulsively could do this to us. When we learned that we couldn't diet compulsively any longer, it set us on a whole new path of living.

God, I pray for the health and well-being of those in recovery. I pray for my own health and well-being.

FOR TODAY: Health and well-being are my standards.

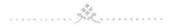

AVOIDING FURTHER SUFFERING   APRIL 24

"Help us to put behind - the plaguing fears, the nagging guilt, the remorse - those things that haunt us year after year."
--Kenneth O. Jones, Minister & Writer

 voiding further suffering seems like a good plan.

FOR TODAY: It is Spring. The flowers are blooming. They have come up out of the cold earth. The sun has warmed the earth. I take a lesson from the sun, and am warm to myself.

ew growth begins in the cold and dark of April.

My experience will no longer be founded on a chemically altered view of reality. New memories will come. I can receive tenderness. It is genuinely given. I receive it genuinely. I don't have to earn or deserve it because of weight loss.

FOR TODAY: I give the perfect sublime smile to someone I know who may not be expecting it. A kind loving smile to a stranger will give me pleasure. I think of myself in a loving kind way. I am a person able to give something of value to another.

"Our spiritual and emotional growth in A.A. does not depend so deeply upon success as it does upon our failures and setbacks. If you will bear this in mind, I think you will see your slip will have the effect of kicking you upstairs instead of downstairs."
        --As Bill Sees It, Alcoholics Anonymous

e may have become enchanted with a new trigger food, diet product or method. We try it. This confirms that we do not have as much control as we thought we did. It may prove again that the food or substance or method isn't an answer, but rather a symptom of our afflicted thinking. We need a Power greater than ourselves for growth.

FOR TODAY: I can recognize trying another trigger food or dieting product as a slip, rather than as an appropriate behavior. This recognition is spiritual progress for me.

I may have felt I deserved punishment, rather than kindness. Working through my fear and desperation builds self-esteem. Letting go of "diethead" and "punishment head", I am aware of and no longer practice these punishment cycles.

FOR TODAY: I select activities that are kind to me. I practice kindness. I make sound choices about kind behavior, kind words, and kind self-thought. I get out the feather.

"Bullying is the act of intentionally causing harm to others, through verbal harassment, physical assault, or other more subtle methods of coercion such as manipulation....Bullying is an act of repeated aggressive behavior in order to intentionally hurt another person, physically or mentally....The effects of bullying can be serious and even fatal....Bullying can also be used as a tool to conceal and boost self esteem: by demeaning others, the abuser him/herself feels empowered....There are other risk factors such as quickness to anger and use of force, addiction to aggressive behaviors, mistaking others' actions as hostile, concern with preserving self image, and engaging in obsessive or rigid actions." --Wikipedia

We all know the difference between receiving tenderness and being bullied. We all know when, and where, and by whom, we are allowed to be safe for who and as we are. Now if we translate this, we can ask -- how do we treat ourselves?

FOR TODAY: Recognizing bullying as part of what has happened, I go forward with a new awareness. I translate that awareness into positive actions to see coercion and bulleying is not permitted by me or others. I know the difference between receiving tenderness and being bullied.

"My great willful wishful acts to lose weight any way possible, as the apex goal of perfectionism, kept me climbing the evil mountain. Making up diets as I went, climbing, sliding back, hounded by evil screaming monkeys, getting degrees of education, certificates of worth, as I climbed...A male angel picked me up and brought me back to earth." --Anonymous

Many of our stories are too real, too frightening to tell without the guilded veil of metaphor or story. There is horror. There is a happy ending. The great stories in the world tell of heroism, trial, safe guardians, making new discoveries about ourselves. All those elements are in our personal stories. We are still living them.

FOR TODAY: I take my own story with me. I am still creating it.

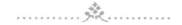

eceiving Tenderness in Illness - I am moved emotionally and I am grateful.

I will use today to remember those people who have shown a special tenderness and kindness for me in the winding paths, gulleys, and brambles, of my affliction. I am grateful today to be in recovery. I never wanted to harm or hurt others or have them worry or stress about me when I was dieting compulsively. I never wanted to have my behavior and abilities to be responsive in life limited by "diethead." I never wanted to cause others suffering.

God, I give thanks for my loved ones and dear friends, who have blessed me with nurture and confidence and love. They live in my heart. I give thanks for their tenderness and their encouragement in times of sickness. I am sensitive to their emotional responses during times of trouble with compulsive eating and compulsive dieting. I am sensitive to how their kindness and the blessings of my continued survival lead me to new growth. I have an increased kindness toward myself and others in the world.

For Today: I live and learn in the lessons of kindness.

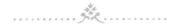

"I don't know where to begin. There are so many things that are untrue. I heard and thought that my life would be ruined if I was one inch to many inches fat. Not true. I was told that diet pills would solve my problem with weight. Not true. Diet remedies created problems with my thinking that other people who were not taking diet remedies didn't have. I thought that compulsively dieting would be an answer to the problems of living. Not true."
                                                        --Anonymous

So many lies. Where to begin? What we were taught? What we were told? What we bought into? Self-deception? Deception of others? Fears of being fat? Fears of what being fat would mean? What we believed about sizes and scale numbers and the people who had them? What we believed about the control we would have over food through diet substances and compulsive dieting? Facing some of the lies and faulty beliefs – because I have to – I can open the door to personal truths.

Letting go of compulsive eating and the compulsive dieting is about living in self-truth because I have to. For me, if I do not let go of eating compulsively and dieting compulsively I continue in illness and impaired thinking.

FOR TODAY: I meditate on truth.

"There is a truth which is of Satan. It's essence is that under the semblance of truth it denies everything that is real. It lives upon hatred of the real and the world which is created and loved by God. It pretends to be executing the judgment of God upon the fall of the real. God's truth judges created things out of love, and Satan's truth judges them out of envy and hatred."
--Dietrich Bonhoffer, Minister & Writer

Going from childhood to adolescence to maturity to young adulthood to middle age, to middle middle age, and older, the body will change many times. Yet we panic in all these changes. We try to deny the changes, the growth, the shape, the new person we are becoming. We want to self-stop. We want to deny the real.

Our culture places much emphasis on denying the real, rather than acknowledging or praising it. The popular culture promotes products and behaviors to stunt growth, to speed up growth, to mask the real, to alter the real. I need to ask myself if my behaviors are hating the real.

FOR TODAY: I strive to love created things.

"I looked again at the pictures of the child. I was that child. I was the size and shape and weight in miniature proportion I would be all my life. I was a healthy, normal child." --Anonymous

I n their rush to control, to modify through science, to mold the child plastically, many parents and health practitioners buy into a bogus health issue. They refuse to see the child they've got. They attempt to alter the natural size, shape, weight, set point, fat distribution of the child. They do a horrible injustice to the child they've got. They focus on size rather than the potentials for building identity based on abilities, interests, enthusiasms.

Lord, Let me appreciate parents, caretakers, teachers, and providers who nurtured me and helped me build solid positive identity.

For Today: I practice justice in my love of the real.

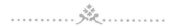

"Where survival alone counts, moral considerations are nearly obliterated.... Terror achieved its most terrible triumph when it succeeded in cutting the moral person off." --Sissela Bok, Writer

T here is a floor beneath which justice and morals do not survive. When my only standard was weight loss any way possible, I lost all conscience or other moral choice.

For Today: My survival does not depend on losing weight or taking diet substances or dieting compulsively. My survival depends on developing life skills, using wise-mind, living by values, living in peace and recovery, living in harmony and interdependence with others.

"A fear that captures our whole attention generates the repetition of negative images and affirmations. It holds within it a power."
                                                        --Anonymous

ear too, instilled in us, can be a lie. "False Evidence Appearing Real." Fear, starting as an emotion that causes fight or flight, can create an exaggerated image or assumption about the world that is false. We deprive ourselves of the newness and excitement of lived experience. Lived life encounters people afresh. It is best to live in real experience, today.

FOR TODAY: I recognize some of the lies instilled in me. I let some of the lies move out and the new perspective move in.

"Most American women think they are winning when they are losing. Jumping on that scale first thing in the morning used to define whether I had a good day. Now success comes from doing the awareness work. I work on my values, my material and my presentation. I work on my food plan and have safety and security all around me. I can show up for rehearsal with no makeup, and people tell me 'You're glowing'." --Anonymous

detach from weight loss as my definition of success and survival. I open up to those abilities and attributes that will, in fact, make me successful in the world. What is my definition of success? Maybe I can define success so that it deals only with today. Perhaps I can define success to be more inclusive of many aspects about myself. Do I define myself only by my successes? If I can forgive myself when I fail at something, maybe that is a successful day.

God, Let me be more inclusive in my definitions of success. We are individual in our successes.

FOR TODAY: Praise and endorsement is kind behavior. Love builds up.

"A Lie is a false statement or piece of information deliberately presented as being true; a falsehood.....It is to this question alone- the intentional manipulation of information - that the court addresses itself in its request for 'the truth, the whole truth, and nothing but the truth.'" --Sissela Bok, Writer

W e want truthful information from health providers in all areas. We want truth in advertising and government regulation of medications. Those in positions of trust should be accountable for information affecting the welfare of others. Yet we know misinformation is transmitted – knowingly or unknowingly. Professionals are often subject to the lobbying efforts of advertisers and their profession. Diagnoses and treatment modalities are often suggested based on misinformation.

Yes, people in authority should not harm others. There are not enough authorities to monitor all the wrongs and injustices in the world. We assume personal responsibility for our individual decisions.

God, I turn my will and my life over to You.

FOR TODAY: I assume personal responsibility for my individual decisions.

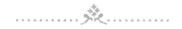

"I was always looking outside myself for strength and confidence but it comes from within. It is there all the time."
--Anna Freud, Children's Psychoanalyst

Claiming my strength is a way of not living in the lie. I am not weak. I don't have to believe a lie – I can discount it. I knock on the door of the Twelve Step rooms and ask for help - my solid foundation. This contradiction, this paradox is level ground. With the help of my Higher Power and others in recovery, I have the strength to discount lies, live in truth, and exert a positive influence on myself and others.

FOR TODAY: I claim my strength. I am able to detach from lies. I must survive today in health. I find confidence in my abilities. I am successful.

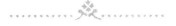

Listening to the voices of the wrong people and jumping to conclusions based on the wrong advice can be disastrous. The messages can be harmful when they incite to the wrong action. All that alarm can cause us to do alarming things, things not thought out.

FOR TODAY: I don't jump at the advertisements about a new weight loss product or method or the packaging that says "eat me" to trigger foods. I separate the voices of alarm and faulty enticements - from the assurances provided by my faith in my Higher Power. My faith in my Higher Power gives me the assurance that I will be able to use wise-mind. For after all, God gave us our minds to use.

"I went to the doctor saying I wanted to lose weight any way possible, no matter what the cost..." --Anonymous

Demanding a quick cure, a relief to my frustration, I may have shut out the hidden costs. I may not have asked, or didn't want to know, the side effects, the long term effects, the demands on my body, or the costs in dollars and cents to contine taking a substance or cure. It is hubris or pride to demand a quick cure to my frustration, at the cost of my body. I didn't create myself. Why should I think that I can make all-powerful demands of myself.

FOR TODAY: Living on the basis of unsatisfied demands will make me miserable. I question myself when I start to make demands, or shut out unpleasant or hidden facts about what I am demanding.

"I have played 'cafeteria doctor' by self-diagnosing." –Anonymous

Lying to ourselves and to our doctors, we contribute to problems. If we have self-diagnosed, and gone to the doctor saying we want diet pills, we have played "cafeteria doctor". Most of us are not licensed M.D.s. The doctor may have prescribed diet pills, covering up another condition, instead of evaluating our health. A "cafeteria doctor" is someone who casually diagnoses friends and family as in a cafeteria (or on an elevator, as in 'elevator lawyer') or someone who self-diagnoses or advises others saying take one of this and one of that as in a cafeteria .

FOR TODAY: I am active in my healthcare. I can be honest with my healthcare providers. I am not in false control by withholding information, or by telling a provider what to do. I am responsible for my decisions.

SO MANY LIES

"We who are your closest friends feel the time has come to tell you that every Thursday we have been meeting, to devise ways to keep you in perpetual uncertainty, frustration, discontent and torture, by neither loving you as much as you want nor cutting you adrift." –Philip Lopate, Poet

rigger foods and foods calling us to ear "more" are not our friends. Diet pills or compulsive dieting methods are neither our trusty friends, as we would like to believe, or our saviors. Duplicity can take many forms. The lies may be enticing and colorful. Yet, we must look foremost to ourselves. Compulsive eating and dieting compulsively kept us in there while delivering frustration, discontent and torture. It is our choice to detach.

FOR TODAY: I look to myself to see who is my real friend and who isn't. I watch what they do and how they behave. I keep a keen eye on people, places and things, while I guide my ship with the lights from my Higher Power and trusted members of the Twelve Step Recovery programs.

"I wore rhinestone glasses from the five and dime, with rosey colored lenses, and went tripping through the fields of naivete, picking and chewing the field daisies that said 'eat me. you will lose weight.' The safe guardians watched over me and guided me away from that field before gently removing those glasses. "
                                        --Anonymous

A llowing myself to be deceived, I have believed what I wanted to. Wishes in a box. Keeping blinders on for as long as I could, I shut out that part of me that was adult, sober, more truthful.

FOR TODAY: Today I decide what is important and where I am going to put my energy. I chart my course in life - to live well each precious day.

- - - - - - - - - - - - - 🏹 - - - - - - - - - - - -

"I drink diet sodas and take diet products. Then I binge on birthday party food, things people bring in to the teacher's lounge, and fast food." --Anonymous.

I t is inconvenient to face the most banal truths about eating choices and behaviors. Yet, facing inconvenient facts is part of living in truth. It is important to not deceive ourselves with vagueness about food and behavior.

FOR TODAY: Taking extra time to meditate on my choices and behaviors - just observing - gives me new information.

PUTTING OUR LIVES ON THE BASIS OF TRUTH
MAY 15

"We must be entirely honest with somebody if we expect to live long or happily in this world....We pocket our pride and go to it, illuminating every twist of character, every dark cranny of the past. Once we have taken this step, withholding nothing, we are delighted. We can look the world in the eye. We can be alone at perfect peace and ease. Our fears fall from us. We begin to feel the nearness of our Creator.... we ask if we have omitted anything, for we are building an arch through which we shall walk a free man at last. Is our work solid so far? Are the stones properly in place? Have we skimped on the cement put into the foundation? Have we tried to make mortar without sand?"
                --*Alcoholics Anonymous*, Third Edition

When regard for truth has been broken down or even slightly weakened, all things will remain doubtful. We need to put our lives on the basis of truth.

I confide in another trusted human being. Confiding does not harm ourselves or others. We do not need to lug along past behavior in every present conversation or relationship. Our past has a value because it brought us closer to our Higher Power and others. Our lives continue to unfold with divine care and direction.

Putting my life on the basis of truth, I admit I don't have the control I once thought I did over food. I have daily opportunities to look at the truth, faulty thinking or shortcomings – self-condemnation, anger, avoidance, being prideful, or acting out of wishful desire. I can decide to start praising instead of condeming - finding the good. I can let go of isolation and self-centeredness instead of going it alone.

FOR TODAY: I put my life on the basis of truth. I help others because I recognize the true. I let go of self-deceptions and naively allowing myself to be deceived by others.

"The crucial difficulty is precisely, I think, that deception is so easy." --G.J. Warnock, Writer

When I have used food, substances or compulsive dieting to create a chemically induced high, in other words as an "energy booster," I have entered a whole other realm of deception. Deceiving others and abusing myself with "energy boosters" and chemically-induced highs doesn't feel very good. It is based on a lie, and a fear that I am not good enough.

If I am using food to "narcotize" I am not facing my problems or am depressing myself and avoiding a fullness of life I can create with my Higher Power and the Twelve Step fellowship.

If I am not functioning well as I am, I need to assess many things. I may need to assess what I am functioning at, my jobs, my roles, the requirements of my job and my roles and what I require of myself. The important thing is to not play 'cafeteria doctor' and self-medicate with trigger foods, diet substances or other substances. I need to talk with my care providers.

God, I pray for wisdom and discernment to make all the changes and adaptations I will need to make as I go through life and make decisions.

FOR TODAY: I go where the love is. I choose a job that is a good fit. There I can make an authentic contribution.

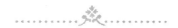

"Most of our platitudes notwithstanding, self-deception remains the most difficult deception. The tricks that work on others count for nothing in that very well-lit back alley where one keeps assignations with oneself: no winning smiles will do here..."
--Joan Didion, Writer

I have tricked myself about what I have needed to do. I need to accept myself as a real flesh and blood human being, deal with overeating or undereating, accept my body changes, deal with life issues such as getting a livelihood, entering the world, risking intimacy, developing relationships, being useful.

I have tricked others. I have maintained secrets. I have entered into relationships with food and diet secrets. I have been inclined to carve out my egotistical willful wishes. Maintaining secrets and deception sometimes seemed an answer and may have worked for awhile, allowing me to live in my diethead of fantastic control and possibilities. Perhaps it allowed me to make social and romantic conquests.

The deception started to melt when the behavior started to become a consuming identity in itself. For many of us, it consumed us. The lifesyle failed to meet the requirements of living. For some of us, the deception stumbled and fell when we were made ill from the diet substances and compulsive dieting. For others of us, the deception had to tumble when we realized we were a certain size, shape, body type or weight, and could not change that reality very much, no matter what diet substances we used, for how long, or what compulsive dieting methods we performed – even to the point of physical collapse. We could hold the deception no longer that compulsive dieting would change our basic selves.

God, Please remove my self-deception. It does not provide a sound basis for living.

FOR TODAY: Reality, the fact that I am alive and breathing and have a sound mind looks pretty good.

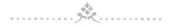

BEING "SMART"– DECEIVING MYSELF   MAY 18

"Intelligence at the service of poor instinct is really dangerous."
–Gloria Steinem, Writer & Activist

We could be assured, dogmatic, and "smart" about food and compulsive dieting methods, and swear to anyone that what we were doing was safe. The messages on TV and radio were equally assured and dogmatic - "Promotes weight loss...," "Not like the others...," "You can lose in 30 days..." As my life became more unmanageable, I have had to question dogmatic authority. Humility looks like a better answer than dogmatism. I have no reason to buy and praise the scientific cure of the latest diet substance. The answers touted by the common culture, are not such good answers for me.

God, Lead me to greater wisdom. It grows out of Your view of me as a precious human being.

FOR TODAY: I am capable of finding meaning and health. I use wise-mind - it is more intelligent than being "smart."

"Hypocrisy means acting on a stage and then acting a part offstage. It assumes a false appearance of virtue or goodness."
--Webster's New World Dictionary

ow I have played the hypocrite. Onstage, using energy boosters, diet boosters or blasters, or central nervous system stimulants allowed me to play act a part. I hid it from teachers, bosses, co-workers, family, and myself. Keeping it offstage allowed me to practice grandiosity and hypocrisy.

FOR TODAY: I am modest. I act with integrity. I enjoy being visible with a single face in the world. I live honestly and like my behavior. I am more open.

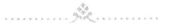

"In the Kingdom of Weight Loss, if I lost a pound, I thought I was nearer the throne. Surely, I deserved more deference, praise, acknowledgement. People should bow down to me."
--Anonymous

any women and men, in all sizes and with various degrees of difficulty or non-difficulty with their weight, play act at being 'holier than thou' – based on weight numbers. I have been drawn into this too. I have believed that, perhaps, people with lower numbers truly were 'holier than thou,' closer to the throne. This is not true. I too have played at being 'holier than thou' when I saw weight loss. Jumping on the scale every two minutes, I thought any weight loss would make me 'holier than thou.'

FOR TODAY: I have a realistic view of other people. I contribute from my individual abilities. I don't headtrip or live in 'The Kingdom of Weight Loss.'

"Most human beings today waste some twenty-five to thirty years of their lives before they break through the actual and conventional lies which surround them." --Isadora Duncan, Dancer

he courage to be yourself with all your moles and imperfections is the beginning to giving up the lies that these things don't exist. It takes courage to look ourselves squarely in the face and say "this I can do; this I can't do."

Whether we wanted to play in an orchestra and see that our career has taken us in another direction, or whether we wanted to be a size 2 and see that our size, shape and body type will never be a size 2, it is important to face our truth at this moment. The conventional lie in our culture is that "you can do anything you want."

FOR TODAY: I go forth accepting and praising what I've got.

LETTING GO OF THE POSE   MAY 22

"Let the world know you as you are, not as you think you should be, because sooner or later, if you are posing, you will forget the pose, and then where are you?" --Fannie Brice, Actress

he pose, the false face we put on, covered up fear. "What will happen when I stop taking diet substances or dieting compulsively?" "What will happen if and when I gain weight from overeating or from my natural body type or heredity?" Whatever we discover will be manageable. These are the Promises of the Twelve Step Program of Recovery, patterned on A.A. We are on the right road. When we turn our lives and our will over to the care of God as we understand Him, and work in fellowship with others, we will discover answers for living without our substance abuse or dieting abuse.

FOR TODAY: I let the world know me as I am. My true identity appears.

So Many Lies

"Media messages said 'You need to lose weight or you will die at an early age.' I thought 'Thin people don't die.' That wasn't true. I got out of my head and got to know people. Once I saw my inborn health, any gloom lifted. I eat right. I take my food from the Greysheet Food Plan. I am very grateful for this body God has given me. --Anonymous

Who has projected images of early death on me? Did these messages contribute to sadness, despair, feelings that I wasn't made right? Why did I believe the messages? Why did I think advertising messages were talking about "me?" Advertisers never met me. Advertisers and family and friends who projected images of early death on me didn't know my genes, or how eating my healthy planned meals over many years would benefit me. I am not a statistic.

Let any gloom I carry lift! Spring is in the air. Let me not react to messages from the media that might drive me to unpredictable behaviors!

FOR TODAY: Let the joyous day begin. I am alive - and alive to it. I have a chance to take good nutrition.

"Left to its own devices, my mind spends much of its time having conversations with people who aren't there."
                                    --Anne Lamott, Writer

e-selfing, by giving our power away to the voices of criticism, is also a form of social lying. We de-self. We people-please. We discount ourselves.

We exist. That is the truth. We do not need to de-self, to pretend that we do not exist. We are real.

FOR TODAY: I exist. I quiet any voices of self-criticism and accept what I've got. I work with what I've got.

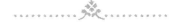

"Oh, that this too too solid flesh, should melt, thaw and resolve itself into a dew." –William Shakespeare, *Hamlet*

eclaiming my own voice requires diligence. Being aware of the paranoia, the internalized messages, the injunctions to do this or do that, I can hardly hear myself at times. Perhaps I need to hear myself express, as Shakespeare did, the burdens of the flesh. The feelings he expresses are so modern. He wrote and identified these feelings over five hundred years ago.

FOR TODAY: Development of a personal voice, with my own truth, is possible.

"Deception is a means to unjust coercion, but also to self-defense and survival." --Sissela Bok, Writer

eeing my humanness is so important. The need for a moral inventory is required when I approach deception. I felt coerced because I was so fearful. I thought my very survival depended on bowing to the coercion. Taking Step Five and admitting to God, to ourselves and to another human being how I was affected gets me closer to the complexities. I harmed myself, I lied to myself, I thought it was a matter of survival to live in the lie and the coercion about what I could do to change my body type, size, shape and weight. There is much unburdening to be done. I take Step Five, identifying who I have harmed, with an experienced Sponsor. Seeing myself with understanding, empathy, consideration is important.

Lord, You offer an ethic of freedom - forgiveness - renewal - and abundant life. I see there is a Higher Power to leading my life.

FOR TODAY: I walk slowly but deliberately toward my goals. I see my humanness.

"The Greek word "krisis" means "discrimination," "judgment," "decision," "crisis," or "trial." It always involves human perception of an unfolding event - a war, an illness, a trial: but it can also sometimes stress the moral element of personal choice which goes along with perception when there is something at stake and opportunity to intervene." --Sissela Bok, Writer

The terror and confusion of "If I don't stop overeating or undereating, I'm going to gain weight or make make myself really sick other ways" competed with "How can I stoP? If I stop it will be painful. How can I handle life?" The terror and confusion of "If I don't take a diet pill or diet compulsively I'm going to gain weight," competed with "If I continue to take a diet substance and diet compulsively it is going to kill me, or take my mind, or put me in the hospital." Both thoughts pushed me closer to the bottom. Crisis led me to make a personal choice, a life choice, a moral choice. It becomes the most moral choice because it chooses the good on which life, true life depends. I may gain or maintain weight. I may lose weight. I will use food in a healthy and planned way with a Sponsor. For me, something is at stake and I have made a decision. I cannot take diet remedies, diet substances or diet compulsively.

God, You and I know my personal choice – I choose life-affirming behavior.

FOR TODAY: I plan my meals ahead of time and turn them over to my Sponsor. I plan where I will get my food. Or I take my prepared meals with me. This preparation takes much of the worry out of my day. This assures me I will be provided for – I have enough and the right food.

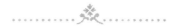

"The very first thing I tell my new students on the first day of a workshop is that good writing is about telling the truth."
                                        -Anne Lamott, Writer

Good living is about living in authenticity. This means acknowledging where I have come from, the messes I have made, what I have tried, and walking on to a better way with realistic expectations, healthy experiences, and practices with real food.

FOR TODAY: I will tell a "story" today that tells the truth. It will contain color, verve, details, emotion, humor perhaps.

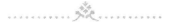

I think of incidences where someone projected a falsehood onto me. My responsibility is to counter falsehoods, first in my own mind, then to correct the other person if necessary. I recognize a falsehood. I don't agree with it. I don't internalize a false projection or statement.

God, You provide safety. You provide intelligence and discernment. Tossed by the winds, I am resilient and well made.

FOR TODAY: I quickly disarm falsehoods.

"Things I never imagined have come into my life." --Anonymous

Finding a balance between "I don't deserve" and "I deserve everything" isn't easy. Neither is true. I have been either self-effacing or arrogant. I have thought either I deserved nothing, or I deserved everything - and you should provide for my every whim and wish. I deserve respect, civil behavior, and justice. I deserve equal opportunities to work and earn a living, to enjoy life, and to contribute to the well-being of others. My realistic expectations of what I deserve are met many times. Other times people don't give me what I deserve - this I recognize and leave it alone or formulate a complaint, because I can take care of myself. If people give me more than I deserve, in generosity, in great good fortune to me, I am extremely happy, and grateful.

For Today: The world is abundant. I let it provide for me. Other people provide for me. I recognize the ways someone gives to me as the way they are able to provide and show love. I receive what is provided and allow the provision and kindness to touch me. I am grateful also for the privacy and freedom I am allowed - when people do not pay attention to me, or interfere, and give me space to live my own life.

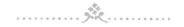

"It is a pleasure to stand upon the shore, and to see the ships upon the sea: a pleasure to stand in the window of a castle, and to see a battle and the adventures thereof below: but no pleasure is comparable to the standing upon the vantage ground of truth (a hill not to be commanded, and where the air is always clear and serene), and to see the errors, and wanderings, and mists, and tempests, in the vale below so always that this prospect be with pity, and not with swelling or pride."

--Francis Bacon, Philosopher

he pleasure of living in truth is empowering. While I may need to claim it quietly, without fanfare, and there may be no party cheering me, it gives a presence and stature no one can take away. Any doubt others may plant in my mind or on my body becomes irrelevant. I know truth that lives on the real. I know truth that affirms the real. When I hear other people talk about diets, dieting methods, clothes fitting or not fitting, sizes, numbers on the scale, what diet they are following, or what diet they just left, I don't have to jump on their bandwagon. I don't have to either be paranoid, thinking they are pointing their conversation at me, or be self-satisfied, because I know they are troubled. I have had and have my own troubles. Yet I know my own truth. I cannot take diet pills, diet herbs, energy boosters, diet blasters, diet blockers, appetite suppressants or other diet substances. I cannot diet compulsively. I am a compulsive overeater. I have a chosen path. I have learned I do not have the control I thought I did over food or diet substances and methods.

God, Thank You for letting me discover the Twelve Steps of Recovery. Thank You for letting me have the wisdom to apply the principles to my troubles.

FOR TODAY: I say five true things about myself. I say five good things that are true about myself. I say five true things that I know. I say five good things that are true about my job, my loved ones, my life.

"Coming to Step 0: I have a moment of clarity. I realize I don't have the control over food I thought I had with diet remedies.
                    --Anonymous

assive dependence on the diet remedy landscape does not work for me.

FOR TODAY: By evaluating and assessing what is true or not true, learning to act on self-truth, and taking wisdom from the countless ages and living tradition, I become a contributor to a life-affirming tradition about letting go of compulsive dieting that will be useful to others.

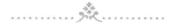

bstaining from compulsive dieting is necessary for me. While the landscape changes, the landscape remains the same -- another day, another brand name, another ingredient or method. The compulsion to try all of them and to continue using them has been great. It is a compulsion that has led nowhere except illness for me. I want to recover from this compulsion. I want to recover mental and physical health. In foolishness, weakness, and hope, I respect my realization. I practice openness to the untried, new ways of thinking, because I need to. I cannot escape life as it is given to me. If I know what it means to be in concert with my Higher Power, I shall know how to use life as it is given to me.

FOR TODAY: I have clarity -- I cannot continue to take diet substances or diet compulsively to deal with compulsive overeating.

have listened intently to the radio and television advertisements about diet substances. I have read labels. I have talked to physicians about ingredients or what would happen. This behavior has been based on interest, hope, as well as, uncertainty, doubt, fear, self-knowledge, knowing the truth about myself as a magic-think diet product substance user before I even asked. I practice abstinence from the products, methods and behaviors. Then I work Steps 1-12 in Twelve Step fellowship to learn more and to get support for life, and overeating and undereating issues.

For Today: I need support. I have clarity.

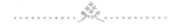

y way of life with abstaining from compulsive dieting, and working a Twelve Step program of recovery for compulsive overeating, one day at a time, is a way of healing for me. I cannot decide for another. I practice my recovery.

God, Accept me and this life-affirming path I have chosen. It is necessary for my health and well-being and usefulness in the world.

For Today: I keep the focus on myself. I don't decide for anyone else what they should do.

"It is hard to know where it happened. Compulsive dieting became more the cause of problems than the cure."
                              --Anonymous

I have enough problems, naturally, normally, as part of living, without creating problems. I often want to side-step problems, in order to forget about them. Creating new problems becomes an escape. Coming to Step 0 opens the door to something other than dieting compulsively. It opens the door to life, to other interests. It allows me the freedom to continue to build on an identity. It is a new opportunity, as well as hard work, and permits me to focus on what is right with me.

FOR TODAY: Everyday problems are managable. I won't create new problems.

"In a Spiritual Listening Workshop the chaplain said 'Find a scar on your body and tell about it.' I recalled a small scar on the inner mound of my right hand. I was subletting a filmmaker friend's loft for the summer when a tomcat got in the loft. I tried to separate it from my friend's cat. The tomcat bit my hand. I went to go to an infirmary on Spring Street to get stitches."
                              --Anonymous

What do I really know about myself? Some of the smallest details are written into my body. I may have temporarily forgotten them.

FOR TODAY: My body speaks to me with vivid tales of good times and bad. Not dialing pain, I turn away from painful thoughts, self-criticism, "poor-me", "why me" thoughts, and troubled striving. I meditate on how I am cared for, past successes, how I am a good person, and how I am strong.

COMING TO STEP 0

ho can make the decision about giving up diet products and methods as a starting point for dealing with compulsive overeating? Only with my Higher Power, and especially with my Higher Power, will I know that Step 0 is the beginning. It is the beginning of wanting to care for myself and a more inclusive identity and purpose for me. Greater mental and emotional and physical stability will result. Strength will come from my conscious contact with my Higher Power. I will be able to live in health, to be restored to sanity, to live life on life's terms, to make spiritual progress, to help others, and to experience the joy of living.

God, I pray for wisdom, understanding and guidance. I pray to develop my conscious contact with You, my HP, for what is good for me individually.

FOR TODAY: I remember that moment of clarity that brought me to Today. I concede to my innermost self my decision to take Step 0.

"Don't Push the River' is a book I keep on my shelf. It has a picture of an older woman on the cover, the author. I got the book many years ago. I keep it there. I love the title and the wisdom contained in the title. It reminds me about a moment of crisis where I hit bottom and came into O.A." --Anonymous

oming to Step 0 is more than hitting bottom with desperation. It is that moment of clarity when I realize I can't grow up faster than I can, achieve more than I can achieve at the moment, see around the corner at the moment, live the next moment right now, or push the river. I cannot live on self-propulsion.

FOR TODAY: I trust time and process. I trust growth.

"Freedom's just another word for nothing left to lose..."
    --Janis Joplin, Singer-Songwriter

reedom isn't just another word. It is the ability to take the liberty to turn away at a critical moment. Not losing the rest of my life can be bought at the bottom or anywhere on the way up from the bottom.

FOR TODAY: Taking the liberty to be conscious of my condition is responsible. I need to get out of the road. I take the risk to get on another path.

"The pressures to lose weight any way possible are so great in my culture. I almost killed myself succumbing to the pressures. The will to live must have turned me toward the light and given me the clarity to stop." --Anonymous.

he 'will to live' is a psychological force to fight for survival. Psychologists write about the 'will to live' experienced by some survivors in the most dire circumstances in the Nazi concentration camps. The will to live kept them alive.

People with terminal illness often fight for survival based on their will to live.

The quality of how I live, and the choice I make to live, extends my life.

FOR TODAY: I walk lightly on new precious ground.

Receiving the "Gift of Desperation" - G.O.D.

he Gift of Desperation - G.O.D. - has been given to me. It is an awakening. I cannot continue to take diet substances or to compulsively overeat.

FOR TODAY: The "Gift of Desperation" - G.O.D. is a true gift. Coming to Step 0 is my starting point.

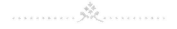

CHOOSING   JUNE 12

"Freedom is often choosing between a rock and a hard place, between the devil and the deep blue sea, between the worst and the less worse. Choosing may involve despair. The loving arms of God are wide and provide perspectives beyond despair."
                                        --Anonymous

e have the freedom to despair, too. By choosing to give up trigger foods, grazing, eating between meals, and excess amounts, we are making that leap of faith into the unknown -- the new, new behavior..

Despair and hopelessness may be an outlook both on continuing to take compulsively diet and overeat and on giving up the behaviors. Despair, however, is likely to be a non-permanent condition. I will choose and widen my perspective.

God, help me. You have given me tremendous freedom, even as I shake in my boots and despair. Help me. Help me take the next steps.

FOR TODAY: I choose a direction. I walk in that direction, trusting I will be supported.

T he need to take "Good Orderly Direction" - G.O.D is a saying coined in Twelve Step Recovery programs.

God, You are a God of the real and not of the abstract. It is a relief to take "Good Orderly Direction." I draw on a greater wisdom. I am not so willful or so isolated.

FOR TODAY: I choose to live. I choose life, to be a flesh and blood person, to not live in my head only, or in my willful wishes.

TRAVELING THE ROAD - HAVING A DIRECTION   JUNE 14

"'Where does this road take me?' someone asked.   'This road doesn't take you anywhere - it's not a traveling escalator you ride on that carries you. You have to be going someplace.'"
--Roland Purdue, Minister

W anting to care for myself and making that decision, puts me on the road to going somewhere. I have to be aware and take actions. I can't be passive. My mental, emotional and physical health, short term and long term, depends on it.

FOR TODAY: "I am responsible". It means I am aware today. I know what road I am on and where I am going for today.

"I doubt myself when others brag about their weight loss. 'Are they the example?' 'Are they the winner?' What are they doing? What are they using?" --Anonymous

I have had a moment of sanity. I realize I can no longer take diet products to deal with compulsive overeating. I will remember what I used to be like, what happened, and what I am like now. I remember my frenzy, my desperation, my doubts about continuing, and what other punishing experiences brought me to Twelve Step Recovery.

FOR TODAY: I am in the right place for me. When I am reading these meditations, or in a meeting, or talking with my Twelve Step Sponsor, my path is clear. I can only take my path.

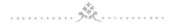

"The good thing about getting older is that you don't lose all the other ages." --Madeline L'Engel, Writer

No matter what age or stage in recovery, I remember other ages or stages where I was using diet products and methods to deal with compulsive overeating. The names on the market and the brand names on the shelves may change. The layers of desperation, fear, self-deception, desire, are vividly recalled, along with more experience, reality testing, and realistic expectations of myself and life.

God, Help me at all my ages. My struggles are real at all ages. Bring me to intelligence, wisdom, right instinct, right caring about my issues and struggles.

FOR TODAY: I won't pretend that I am so "smart" that I can go it alone. I need input from others who know me and care.

"Today I celebrate my anniversary. I have been abstinent from diet remedies and compulsive overeating this year. I value my clear mind. I follow a food plan and program of recovery for right use of food. My blood pressure, cholesterol and blood sugar are normal." --Anonymous

L ong-term health is desirable. Abstaining is a way of healing for me. With abstinence, I can focus on food planning and eating the right foods in the right amounts. I want long healthy life.

FOR TODAY: Life is beautiful. Releasing any despair, I have an opportunity to live a new way. Putting one foot in front of the other, abstinent, I create the health today that will play into tomorrow.

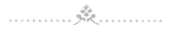

"If you have made mistakes, even serious ones, there is always another chance for you. What we call failure is not the falling down, but the staying down." --Mary Pickford, Actress

H ave you ever seen a person who had to learn to get up from the floor or chair a different way, because they were injured? That's the way I am. I can't get up the same way, because I have been injured by compulsive behaviors. I must learn a new way to get up. Fortunately, the human mind is creative. It creates ways to survive and adapt. Learning from my injuries, I now use the tools of recovery to address diethead thinking and behaving.

God, Help me to acknowledge my handicaps, my bruises, my regrets; take my hurts and teach me a new way, stronger, more stable than the ways I was using.

FOR TODAY: I get up a new way.

COMING TO STEP 0

"I looked at my hands to see if I was the same person now I was free. There was such a glory over everything, the sun came like gold through the trees, and over the fields, and I felt like I was in heaven....I had crossed the line of which I had so long been dreaming. I was free; but there was no one to welcome me to the land of freedom, I was a stranger in a strange land, and my home after all was down in the old cabin quarter, with the old folks, and my brothers and sisters. But to this solemn resolution I came; I was free, and they should be free also; I would make a home for them in the North, and the Lord helping me, I would bring them all there. Oh, how I prayed then, lying all alone on the cold, damp ground; 'Oh, dear Lord,' I said, 'I ain't got no friend but you. Come to my help, Lord, for I'm in trouble!'
--Harriet Tubman, Abolitionist

Coming to Step 0 can be daunting, entering totally new territory, seemingly alone. Coming to an awareness I can no longer continue to take any diet substances or diet compulsively doesn't bring cheers in my culture. There are those who promote the use or sell diet substances and those who use them. There are new methods for dieting compulsively promoted all the time. Stepping into this new territory I receive plenty enough - - first my very survival, recovery from illness, then clarity, then stabilizing mental and physical health. These are visible cheers, witnessed in my well-being. Then long-term health is possible.

God of grace, who constantly brings us to new beginnings and larger possibilities, guide me.

FOR TODAY: I listen to the silence of the question: who ever heard of not dieting or eating compulsively? I hear the loudness of the cheers: millions of men and women in many places and times have lived healthy lives not taking diet remedies to deal with compulsive overeating.

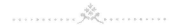

"Creative minds have always been known to survive any kind of bad training." --Anna Freud, Children's Psychoanalyst

L etting go of ineffective coping mechanisms takes courage. Prospering in health is the reward. Why does it take courage? How am I going to deal without what I know? What will happen; what if I'm not in the diet club anymore or going to the diet vendors? Will I be more of an outsider? What if I don't network with other women talking diethead? What will I do with myself? How will I distract myself from my anxiety? How can I go against the 'experts' I've listened to and the messages I've heard; how do I deal with the fear of defying the common culture? How will I reach out to others? What will I do with my time and thinking if I'm not putting it into diethead? What will I do when I get uncomfortable with feelings of self-loathing or lack of self esteem and am in despair about changing myself to be sexier, prettier, younger? What will I do when a new method of dieting compulsively comes out on the market? How will I feel safe in the world if I'm not distracting myself, or punishing myself with food, and defending myself by proving to myself and others that I'm suffering by doing extreme diet?

There will be questions. When I accept this, I won't be so alarmed when they come up. The answers will come. Being uncomfortable and having uncomfortable feelings is not bad.

God, You are my Higher Power. I seek wise counsel. My unhealthy coping mechanisms have come from bad training and were self-selected in earlier times. You are the God of Renewal. You are the God of Growth. After dark times, times of illness, bring me renewal.

FOR TODAY: Because I have a creative mind and because my Higher Power is creative, I am renewed. New windows and doors appear where before there were walls.

I don't have to answer all the questions or solve all my problems at once. I don't have to stress about possible problems. I can set my troubles on the shelf. When I need to address them, I can take them down one at a time, to look at each one more clearly.

I trust whatever may come. I trust because I know that Step 0, my realization, and my decision, are primary. I come into Twelve Step Recovery because I trust there are answers to be learned. I have a Higher Power and a fellowship of people recovering from similar afflictions who will help me walk a happier healthier road.

FOR TODAY: I practice trust in my Higher Power & the fellowship and the tools of recovery.

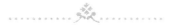

BUILDING NEW MUSCLES - BREAKING ENERGY   JUNE 22

"The mountain creates the wolf. It is the hardship that creates the wolves to survive to another generation. It is hardship for me too, to make the effort to live without diet remedies. The effort builds new and different muscles. It is based on an honest and true awareness of the diet and food environment around me, and what I am doing with food uncovered, no cover-ups. I deal with my real body and metabolism. New lessons open a door about reality."
--Anonymous

Because I take Step 0 , ever so slowly an energy appears. I have clarity of what is important to me. I want to continue to build my identity based on my God-given talents, abilities and enthusiasms.

FOR TODAY: I trust answers will come in the hard work of living. I focus on what is right with me. The mountain creates the wolf. While it may be difficult, there is satisfaction in the effort.

"Meeting myself at Step 0 is like meeting myself at Ground Zero. I never want to face that catastrophe again. I am terribly afraid of collapse from dieting compulsively. You lived through this horror, I say to myself. Claim it. You can take the next thing that comes along." --Anonymous

Step 0 appeared in my life because I was ready for it. I was not spiritually teachable until my illness forced me to look in that direction. It was all that was left; no human power could relieve my compulsion to use diet remedies and methods to deal with compulsive overeating. Putting Step 0 first means I recognize the thinking and fears that led me to diet compulsively and overeat compulsively. I have clarity. I cannot continue these behaviors.

FOR TODAY: I am healthy with a sound mind. This is important to me. I want health and well-being.

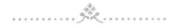

Whether I have had a low bottom, or a higher bottom, it is not a competition.

FOR TODAY: I want recovery from use of diet substances and compulsive dieting for myself. I want health for you. I want it for myself.

utting Step 0 first, means putting down the diet substances and compulsive dieting and dealing with food issues.

I value my abstinence from compulsive overeating and from diet products and methods as much as an alcoholic values his or her sobriety. I see the importance of this abstinence. My illness is about more than just not taking the diet remedies, dieting compulsively, or losing weight. It is about more, the same way the alcoholic's illness is about more than just not drinking alcohol. I come into Twelve Step Recovery to be relieved of my compulsion and unworkable attitudes toward living.

FOR TODAY: I take Step 0. In Twelve Step meetings, I discover more about the nature of my problems. Step 0 has appeared in my life because I am ready for it. I am glad today for it.

NOURISHING STRENGTH JUNE 26

"Everything nourishes what is strong already."
--Joan Didion, Writer

 appily, I am strong. My moment of clarity grows in proportion to my desire to live and my positive evaluation of my resilience and ability to move forward in health and renewal. Because I have tremendous hope for a wonderful life, I want to preserve that life in its best form. I don't want to go slinking around trying to be somebody else. This is the truth.

God, You made me strong.

FOR TODAY: The summer trees are in their full glory. The branches are strong holding up the leaves to absorb the sun. I take time to take in the beauty. I know and enjoy the fact that I am strong.

I accept my choices and my decisions, including any sacrifices that may result from not overeating, for the better life I have chosen.

The alcoholic might think they would function better with a drink. I might have a passing thought that I would function better at a lower weight. I might think I need to lose 10 pounds for a wedding or reunion, and I will take just one month of substances, or one year. I might have a sudden desperation, triggered by anything., to try a new trigger food or diet remedy. I might have a desperate fear of body changes or weight gain or weight numbers. However, considering the cost, in possible return to uncontrolled diethead, self condemnation, and the illness that resulted for me, Step 0 allows me to keep that moment of clarity in front of me, when I realized I could no longer continue to diet compulsively. Not practicing methods of compulsive dieting is a sacrifice I willingly make. I can't buy this kind of sanity.

FOR TODAY: I choose a better life by not compounding problems.

"I never lose an opportunity of urging a practical beginning, however small. For it is wonderful how often a mustard seed germinates and roots itself." --Florence Nightingale, British Nurse

Coming to Step 0 is a practical beginning. A moment of sanity has led me to a new path. I strive for freedom. This is my starting point for nursing myself to health. I believe I cannot come to a wholesome and healthy life until I address my afflictions..

FOR TODAY: I make a practical beginning.

"Be courageous. It's one of the only places left uncrowded."
   --Anita Roddick, The Body Shop Entrepreneur

ourage is the price I must pay for going forward. It is not a courage I have chosen lightly. It is a courage that chose me, because it was required for me to live. Hemingway wrote, 'Staring down the face of a charging tiger, he discovered courage.' With my back up against the wall, because the behavior was punishing, disillusioning and created illness for me, I have realized I cannot continue diet and binge cycles or compulsive dieting as a mask for compulsive overeating.

Who would have thought I was heading into unpopulated territory. Others, operating on TV, radio, and magazine ads, and drug store shelves, are focusing on weight loss in ways they have chosen. I do what I have to do and take only my path. I believe I can be relieved of compulsive eating without the use of diet substances or compulsive dieting.

God, You give me courage. You protect me and give me strength.

FOR TODAY: I have confidence. Courage is with me. I call on it as needed. I make decisions and operate on them with the help of my Higher Power.

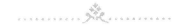

I have tried many things: not eating, liquid fasts, appetite suppressants, central nervous system stimulants, diet boosters, diet blasters, diet blockers, metabolizers, diet bitter herbs, diet herbal teas, diet powders, diet liquids, diet pills, diuretics, purging, laxatives, punishing exercise, prescription drugs, over the counter drugs, compulsive exercise or combinations and variations of all of them. They didn't address my food behavior or my life and living issues. They didn't talk to my spirit or ask that I live on a spiritual level. They didn't address my need for a Power greater than myself.

I believe I can be relieved of compulsive eating without the use of diet substances or compulsive dieting. This hope allows me to have the faith to try the untried. I become willing to search for a spiritual experience. I begin to rely on a Power greater than myself. I believe I can be relieved of my obsession with diet remedies. I separate out my affliction with diet substances and compulsive dieting from issues I may have with compulsive eating. Both are abusive behaviors, but there is a difference. I believe I can be relieved of both abusive behaviors.

FOR TODAY: I go forward one step at a time, knowing one thing is not another. Things are not mixed up in my mind.

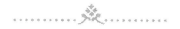

"We admitted we were powerless over food and that our lives had become unmanageable." --Step One, The Twelve Steps
  Adapted by Permission from Alcoholics Anonymous World Services

aking Step One, I let go of control. My attempts to control the physical and the emotional with diet substances and compulsive dieting have failed. I don't understand 'why me'. I don't understand why people are made physically the way they are, in all their shapes and forms. Appearances do not tell an accurate story about the many facets of health. There are people at all sizes, shapes, weight who have good health. There are people at all sizes, shapes, weight who have poor health. Go figure.

A combination of qualities and attributes makes each of us unique, with abilities and limits. I face myself. Scientists touch some of the facts and mystery. We have the mystery and wonder of human generation over millions of years, a combination of genes, nature and nurture, that makes a person a survivor in a particular time, place or habitat from their ancestors.

I don't have to understand everything or try to. Understanding that You, my Higher Power, will me to be and that I can choose survival, health and vitality is enough. I am grateful for what I do understand, through Your Wisdom and the gift of my intelligence.

Today, I ask for help with my addiction. Denial has kept me from seeing how powerless I am and how my life is unmanageable. I need to learn and remember that I have an incurable illness and that abstinence is the only way to deal with it.
  The First Step Prayer, *Alcoholics Anonymous,* Third Edition

FOR TODAY: The mystery and adventure of life are mine. Taking Step One is a beginning. I begin a new learning experience and way of behaving.

I see how I have been smitten with an insane obsession. It could destroy me in the end. I am just as powerless over diethead, and compulsive overeating as the alcoholic over alcohol. Have I not been a victim of a delusion that I could live by self-propulsion and wrest happiness from this world if only I could lose weight? When I fully admit my powerlessness over food and this obsession, I am able to start practicing the remaining eleven steps of Twelve Step Recovery.

FOR TODAY: I stand ready to have this obsession lifted.

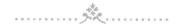

"I thank God for my handicaps, for through them, I have found myself, my work, and my God." --Helen Keller, Activist & Writer

I thought I was omnipotent and could change my body at will to be any size, shape or weight I wanted. My life has become unmanageable because of this obsession. Any life run on denial of the truth can hardly be a success. Limitations are what any of us are inside of. Our limits can be our biggest assets. Our limits help define how we are to develop our talents and meet our challenges. When we start using what we've got, instead of wishing for what we haven't got, then we take up the adventure of living.

FOR TODAY: My limits are my assets. I accept conditions as they are. The remaining eleven steps will show me how to move toward acceptance with dignity and grace. I tap into my Higher Power. New lessons and learning are in store.

The Bill of Rights to the U.S. Constitution, 1789
The First Amendment

"Congress shall make no law respecting an establishment of religion, or prohibiting the free exercise thereof; or abridging the freedom of speech, or of the press; or the right of people peaceably to assemble, and to petition the Government for a redress of grievances."

ndependence Day, July 4th, is a holiday to be celebrated for many reasons. Our nation's leaders took the Liberty to start something new - a new country. Our nation's leaders have laid the foundations of civil and religious liberty.

e can claim the liberty. We can free ourselves from the old insanity.

FOR TODAY: Liberty can be lived quietly every day. It is mine.

LETTING ME IDENTIFY WITH OTHERS   JULY 5

"We admitted we were powerless…" --Step One, The Twelve Steps

e are not alone. I identify. I don't compare. I look for the similarities, not the differences.

God, Let me identify with others, not compare. Even though my pain and my affliction are my own, I begin to understand I am not alone. My painful separation from others begins to subside along with my futile attempts to control expected outcomes. I start living life in fellowship with You and others. I am ready for this moment.

FOR TODAY: I know what it took for me to get here. So I acknowledge your experience with what it took for you to get here too.

"Came to believe a Power greater than ourselves could restore us to sanity." --Step Two, The Twelve Steps

"The word God still aroused a certain antipathy.... My friend suggested what then seemed a novel idea. He said 'Why don't you choose your own conception of God.' That statement hit me hard. It melted the icy intellectual mountain in whose shadow I had lived and shivered many years. I stood in the sunlight at last. It was only a matter of being willing to believe in a Power greater than myself. Nothing more was required for me to make my beginning."
        --Bill's Story, *Alcoholics Anonymous*, Third Edition

W hether you believe in one God, a wisdom built into matter and the operations of life, a wisdom or goodness or Power that exists within each human being, a divine Universe, or a wisdom and direction found within a group, having faith in something bigger and more powerful than ourselves helps us feel safer.

The belief in a Higher Power can help us find meaning and direction. Coming out of extreme isolation or self-centeredness, connecting to our Higher Power can help us open to other facets of ourselves and our being, other than size shape or weight. This connection, relatedness, and discovery can give us hope to find new answers and new happiness. Believing in something divine or holy or "there" to help, whether it be in the Universe, within the Earth or Planet, within us, or the group, can help soothe during distressing emotions or troubling times.

I pray for an open mind so I may come to believe in a Power greater than myself. I pray for humility and the continued opportunity to increase my faith. I don't want to be crazy anymore.
   --The Second Step Prayer, *Alcoholics Anonymous,* Third Edition

FOR TODAY: I write my definition of my Higher Power and what it means to me.

"Hope begins in the dark, the stubborn hope that if you just show up and try to do the right thing, the dawn will come. You wait and watch and work: You don't give up." --Anne Lamott, Writer

"No matter how ruined man and his world may seem to be, and no matter how terrible man's despair may become, as long as he continues to be a man his very humanity continues to tell him that life has a meaning....Our life, as individual persons and as members of a perplexed and struggling race, provokes us with the evidence that it must have a meaning. Part of the meaning still escapes us. Yet our purpose in life is to discover this meaning, and live according to it." --Thomas Merton, Monk & Writer

I come to Twelve Step meetings and listen. I see what other people's understanding of God is. I listen, in humility. I am not in isolation any more. I am free to think for myself, to listen, to evaluate, to discern, to accept that I need to be restored to sanity.

No matter what my state of belief or disbelief or understanding of God, I am willing to discover my meaning. The power to be comes from somewhere. It is mine to use in freedom and responsibility and as I am able to. My humanity speaks. I was made with limits. I will accept those limits. I will live inside those limits and seek to have my life be manageable. I am more than a chemical machine. I am a flesh and blood person.

FOR TODAY: Hope begins in the dark. I lift my head, asking "Is it too late?" I have been told there is hope for a better way. I'm still pretty low to the ground, but I'm unearthed, above ground, vital.

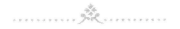

"A loving God -- as I understand God -- is larger than any destruction or evil. A loving God -- as I understand God -- is able to turn around, forgive, protect, or heal from hate or harm. In being larger and more giving and more active than anything else, as the Superme Being, Sovereign, Independent, and Independently giving, this HP is always able to provide, to renew, to be a fountain of health and inspiration and wisdom and guidance to me."

                                   --Anonymous

I n the fellowship we find others who have suffered despair, cynicism, and disappointment. It takes what it takes to recover.

I come to believe I will find a willingness to drop the cynicism and disappointment even though it may come up again. I begin to accept myself as a flesh and blood human being.

FOR TODAY: I celebrate this God-sense. In my darkest hours, in my ugliest self-loathing, in my keenest resentment, or my most hateful aversion to where I am at the moment, I know this God-sense is also there.

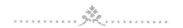

Human beings are a great resource, much better than a substance for solving problems. In sharing, I am relieved of some of my burdens. My experience helps others. Since God often speaks through other people, their experience, strength and hope helps me.

FOR TODAY: My load is lighter because it is shared. It is my responsibility to act. I act with new support and new wisdom.

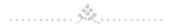

Medical and healthcare practioners could only help me from their perspective. They could not help from the perspective of someone inside the behavior. I become willing to be helped by others like me. God speaks through other people. Being helped by others like me draws on a university of experience, a universe of experience and recovery. We seek to be on the beam and to be on the beam to help others.

FOR TODAY: Peace is with me. When there is an unsettling of the waters, or my feathers are ruffled, or there is a monster in the road that looks mean, I seek a Power greater than myself for help, often in the guiding loving perspective available from another trusted human being.

W e recognize that the care of God may come through other people, especially healthcare practitioners. We pray that caregivers in the healing professions be God's agents. We are grateful for all the caregiving deeds done on our behalf. Both our willingness to seek and accept care, and the availability of people who care and provide good direction, are gifts from our Higher Power.

My experience with food and diet, while personal to me, has been seen by healthcare practitioners in others. I am not terminally unique. Thank God, I am not "terminal" either. I am not dying or dead. I have been blind. Now I let others see me as I am. I learn from what they have seen and learned. I assume responsibility for my care choices. I let myself be cared for.

We pray with thanks for all the caregiving deeds done on our behalf, so our lives may function in health. We pray with appreciation for those who minister to us in the healing professions. We pray in appreciation for those who minister to us to build our identities and abilities by fostering development of our talents in business, in scientific pursuits, in music, art, drama, education, parenting, and career.

FOR TODAY: I have appreciation for care. I recall with a smile those special people and ways those people show their care.

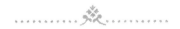

W hether we have gone to a public hospital in emergency to be taken care of, to a medical doctor or psychiatrist in emergency, to a treatment facility, to a loving friend or family member indicating something is wrong, or have come to that knowledge ourselves and have not had an emergency, accepting care may be a needed relinquishment of control and self-will. We let someone else care for us. Taking Steps Two and Three can be a continuation of accepting care. We put aside our false pride. We let down the false fronts.

FOR TODAY: I accept caring.

Thinking sanely means being open to the fullness of life.

M any of us have done the weight control measures. We have thought about every method sold, or prescribed. The single-mindedness of our thoughts has shown us that we did not stop thinking about them, even when "dry." We wanted control of something. It has made me feel empowered. It has distracted me from other life functions. While it was originally an attempt to deal with anxiety, the consuming anxiety it created robbed me of ambition. The anxiety it bred filled the mind to overflowing and washed away any ambition that was not related to losing weight.

Being restored to sanity, "soundness of mind" comes gradually. We are restored to physical and mental health. We practice self-care, build on identity and live manageably a day at a time.

For Today: I want the promises. I seek the fullness of life and freedom from obsession.

*"Somehow I thought I lost the right to eat. That was insanity.
I recognize the insanity now."* --Anonymous

All of us have overheard others talk about their latest diet, how many grams of this or that a food had in it. These people were deciding if they had the right to eat again. I have been caught up in it too.

I rediscover my human rights.

FOR TODAY: Recognition - Enlightenment - Wisdom - Self-knowledge - Faith - Trust - Higher Power - a Twelve Step program with Sponsor, Food Plan - A.A. Literature, Meetings - Telephone - Service. All of these are stabilizing forces. They give me a stability no food or diet remedy can give me.

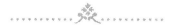

RESIGNING FROM THE DEBATING SOCIETY   JULY 15

I stop fighting anybody or anything. This includes fighting to change things about myself. Fighting gets me nowhere. Cruel action, willful action, ego driven action only bullies me or others around me. Mindful action in concert with my Higher Power brings me "good orderly direction."

FOR TODAY: I care deeply about my real self. I am willing to behave positively, confidently. I am willing to have self-respect. No matter what someone else thinks I should be doing or ways they might offer to know what is best for me, I live in clarity about myself.

"A radical, root change happened in giving up my self-will. I had to get off the wrong train." --Anonymous

Being an adult is a slow becoming based on trying to last and not be snuffed out in a blaze of stupid activity. Getting off the wrong train, by giving up the self-will with compulsive overeating and compulsive dieting, is a good start. Building identity is an arduous process, a process that takes years. People put their energies into their identifications, their choices, their purposes, and build an identity gradually, carefully, arduously. Often there is "slow growth." We want to be on the right train.

FOR TODAY: I want to be true to my identity.

"We made a decision to turn our will and our lives over to the care of God, as we understood Him." -- Step Three, The Twelve Steps

In taking Step Three, I have an awareness that life is a great good and a great gift. I am to enjoy the fullness of life, to self-care, to enhance my looks in pleasurable non-harming ways, to eat healthy food in healthy ways, to build on identity and be in the world.

God, I offer myself to Thee, to build with me and to do with me as Thou wilt. Relieve me of the bondage of self, that I may better do Thy will. Take away my difficulties, that victory over them may bear witness to those I would help of Thy Power, Thy Love, and Thy way of life. May I do Thy will always.
    --The Third Step Prayer, *Alcoholics Anonymous,* Third Edition

FOR TODAY: I access great relief and pleasure in taking the Third Step. I identify my relief and pleasure. I look forward.

When they say "God is in charge," I believe they mean the responsibility doesn't belong to me to control expected outcomes. I am to do what I'm good at and what I like, with my God-given developed talents. It is not my responsibility to fix or run the world or other people.

We all have our Higher Power. Fixing the world or something about "you," is not for me. I am not the 'be all' and the 'end all'.

The responsibility is bigger than me. Recognizing what I am able or not able to do, I live in concert with life as it is given. I recognize what belongs to 'you,' your issues and problems and joys and satisfactions, I can focus on what belongs to 'me.' I am more able to 'respond to' life, situations, other people, and to co-create, co-live, co-solve with my HP when I recognize what part I play and what is mine to do.

FOR TODAY: I live in humility. I don't take on problems that are not mine. I know when something that bothers me is not my fault. I recognize what I can or cannot do.

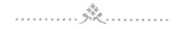

We know that in our individual efforts to control, we have often done the judging. In Step Two *"Came to believe a Power greater than ourselves could restore us to sanity"*, we let go. We observe and then let go of our judgment calls, fault-finding, self-criticism and criticism of others. We seek gut-level wisdom guided by good will.

I observe, just observe, my judgment thoughts, without fault finding in them. I see how many of my thoughts are judgment calls. After watching these thoughts - I let them dissipate. Then I focus on the present moment.

FOR TODAY: I move one grain of sand and the whole beach changes. I release criticism.

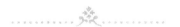

"Thou art the God of sunshine and of clouds, of happiness and of sorrow, of life's times of fulfillment and of the time of reflection and despair....More of our regrets are false and unreal than they are legitimate. O God of new beginnings, help us to hand our spiritual garbage of the past over to Thee for Thy divine disposal in forgiveness." --Kenneth O. Jones, Minister & Writer

Having been spared further self-destruction, I am aware of youth and growing maturity. I am aware of what I cannot do anymore. The Higher Power I understand knows the moods and emotions and behaviors and trials of people. There is Wisdom in this.

When we hand over the garbage of our foolishness, we can walk into a new moment. I get ready to take the Action Steps - Steps Four through Nine. Character defects hurt me. Doing my Fourth Step Inventory lets me know I am not alone anymore. I can give up and over my regrets and claim new practices of love toward myself and others.

For Today: I am willing to let my Higher Power have all of me, to work and walk in greater wisdom.

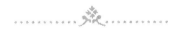

iving the life I have been given, I have an appreciation for the life I have been given and the life that has been preserved.

FOR TODAY: Choosing the lifeforce given me is reason enough to let go of diethead and compulsive overeating, regardless of the pressures or coercion to use or take or practice.

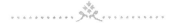

ew energies are released in me because I am not putting my energies into "diethead." My energies are released in a new direction. Recovering in Hope, I build my identity by living, by making sound choices, by thinking mindfully. I realize this energy in "Coming to believe".

I don't have to conquer the world, or be grandiose or prideful. My natural ambition is restored and my drive for constructive satisfaction by focusing on specific, manageable, attainable, realistic pleasures and goals today.

FOR TODAY: I ask what my natural ambitions are for the day. Then I take small steps to realize them. I am hopeful.

"Food is an important part of a balanced diet."
--Fran Lebowitz, Writer

The Twelve Step meetings give me the ground where I can recover the dignity crushed by food and compulsive overeating. All of the Twelve Step suggestions are just that -- suggestions. There are no rules. It is fertile ground in which love and insight can grow. I craved freedom when I first came to Twelve Step meetings, freedom from the bondage of food and the crushing blows of dieting. I have found freedom and warmth. An enduring emotional sobriety and physical recovery is dearly appreciated. I leave regrets outside the gate with the door open; I have passed through the gate.

FOR TODAY: I attend telephone, online chat, and face-to-face Twelve Step meetings.

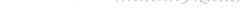

LIVING IN GRATITUDE   JULY 24

"We admitted we were powerless over food and that our lives had become unmanageable." --Step One, The Twelve Steps, Adapted by Permission from A.A.

The key is willingness. When I surrender my will to fix myself my way and claim God's will for me, which is always good, good things happen. The joy of living happens.

God, We offer our praises for the good gift of life, and for the restructuring of our lives.

FOR TODAY: I am grateful. I praise the forces that brought me to this gratitude for new answers.

"To be somebody, you must last." --Ruth Gordon, Actress

y life isn't over. And -- although I may never weigh what I would like to weigh, my possibilities in life are not over. Because overeating and dieting compulsively is not the answer, it's not the end of the world. It's a new beginning.

To be somebody you must last - to grow from your experience and believe in yourself. By making the decision to grow and allow my Higher Power in, in grace and dignity, I receive a great gift I was ready for.

I didn't know that growing would continue for so many years. I look forward to lasting. What I can't change today must be accepted today. I can say "OK God, now what?"

FOR TODAY: I give myself a chance to continue to grow. Each day has 86,400 seconds in it. Each day is filled with myriad sights, sounds, sensations, colors, thoughts, feelings, projects, plans, efforts. My mind and body in recovery can experience, enjoy life, contribute, shape, give direction to, move in positive directions.

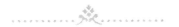

"God, Grant me the Serenity to accept the things I cannot change, the Courage to change the things I can, and the Wisdom to know the difference."
  --The Serenity Prayer, Reinhold Neibuhr, Minister & Writer

S aying "OK God now what?" opens me to the possible, what HP has in store for me and what real talents I can use to meet the environment I live in, what is possible. I don't live on Mars today. I work toward getting and creating a habitat on this earth, with my resources and opportunities. I don't ask for unrealistic resources or opportunities that aren't here on this earth or don't exist. Like a bird, I seek a habitat, which means a place that is livable. I can get food, earn a living, a livelihood, get around, have shelter, occupy a "niche" safely, live in community with others.

FOR TODAY: I move toward my good by using my talents and abilities.

"Sometimes it is enough to put your bedroom slippers on and just be abstinent." --Anonymous

I t is enough to just have the planned meals for the day without diet substances or dieting compulsively. I receive gentleness and tenderness in easing up my drive. People can know my issues with diet substances and compulsive dieting and respect my choices. Spending time with friends and loved ones who support and love me, receiving calls and emails that support me, talking, I receive tenderness.

FOR TODAY: I eat healthy foods and healthy amounts. I have patience and tolerance with myself.

o matter what media personality is advertising a product, or what the claims and justifications are, I am free from the sale. I am safe. I am well. I am protected.

The first freedom I experience is the freedom from diet products and methods. Then I experience the freedom from compulsive overeating. I choose to work on my problems of living. I freely choose to work the Twelve Steps with my Sponsor and the fellowship.

The greatest freedom, for me, is the freedom from doubt. I am free to live in confidence about my awakening. I am no longer dominated by the world and its people.

Life is good. I have a chance to change my perspective. This chance is always available to me. I can learn from others how to walk on brighter paths. I'll see the enchantment of life and I'll share and participate actively.

FOR TODAY: I see the enchantment of life. I share and participate actively.

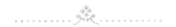

I want to live manageably for the rest of my life. I feel I can do this by taking Steps One, Two, and Three daily.

I am in amazement that I have the prospect of living manageably for the rest of my life. The prospect of living manageably makes working the Twelve Step program worth it. Each day I am grateful for a day of rest from the compulsions of "diethead," and from the low self-esteem caused by my behaviors. Not picking up, buying or using helps create self-esteem. It creates clear thinking and sanity. I move toward giving up the character defects that drove my behavior and caused me trouble. Not using diet products and methods avoids the return of mental or physical illness related to their use or future symptoms. Working a Twelve Step program for eating issues lends a new lease on life. These efforts require work.

There is the pink cloud at the beginning of recovery. There are also the gloomy days of rain and shadow. Each day free of diet products and methods and compulsive overeating builds up in truth and self-esteem. Our zest for life and living makes our decision worthwhile. I am grateful for the gift of life, preservation, health, stability and the joy of living free.

FOR TODAY: Each day free reminds me that I matter.

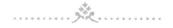

ealing old wounds takes time. I have looked to food and dieting excesses as the instant solution to distress. I have wanted to make sexual conquests. I have wanted to stay in fantasies of control. Growing in understanding takes time. It takes recognizing that I have been wounded. I have been wounded, both by my behaviors and by a society that promotes instant gratification and excessive desire as good. I didn't deserve to be wounded this way. I need to heal.

FOR TODAY: I talk to my Sponsor and others recovering. I have a program of recovery to deal with living. I "Come to believe a Power greater than myself can restore me to sanity."

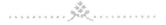

"I don't think that the events of my life are preordained, but they're definitely guided. I hope they're guided because I'd have a [heck] of a time trying to figure it out all by myself!"
                        --Joan Baez, Singer-Songwriter

ife is long. Life is good. Believing that there is support available, we don't have to go it alone. I let down the walls to receive from the world. A baby is born and wouldn't live if it didn't receive support and care. This is the pattern of life. We are part of community and need care whether we want it or not. Believing in support, cooperation and communication is wisdom.

FOR TODAY: I take "Good Orderly Direction" in ways that come from my Higher Power and others.

I n order to stay the course, we have the action steps. The action steps in Twelve Step Recovery -- Steps Four through Nine -- deal with character and values. Taking these steps is a fact finding and fact facing process. It helps us look at our priorities, the use of our instincts, how we have used our resources, and our attitudes towards the causes and conditions in our lives.

"Creation gave us instincts for a purpose. Without them we wouldn't be complete human beings.... So these desires -- for the sex relation, for material and emotional security, and for companionship -- are perfectly necessary, and surely God-given."
--Step Four, *Twelve Steps & Twelve Traditions*

Taking a look can reveal motives in taking diet remedies. Our desires for the sex relation, for material and emotional security, and for companionship are as normal as anyone's. However, our methods of trying to obtain these desires were often wrong-headed, unrealistic or deceitful, when we thought diet substances and compulsive dieting would do the trick.

Desires for control over body size, shape and weight, and achieving control expected outcomes, were unrealistic to life as it is written. Living on the basis of "unsatisfied demands" caused anger, resentment, self-pity and self-absorption.

FOR TODAY: I prepare to write my Fourth Step inventory.

"Made a searching and fearless moral inventory."
   --Step Four, The Twelve Steps

"To state the facts frankly is not to despair the future nor indict the past. The prudent heir takes careful inventory of his legacies and gives a faithful accounting to those whom he owes an obligation of trust."--John F. Kennedy, 35th U.S. President

 here is a need to place my life on a new footing – with new thinking – with new purpose – with new perspective.

I look over my past, the course of my history, and how I have been hurt by attitudes and behaviors. I identify fears, resentments, character defects and shortcomings. Then I am on a better footing to go forward. Models for doing a Fourth Step inventory are available from *The Alcoholics Anonymous Big Book* and the *Twelve Steps & Twelve Traditions.*

A moral inventory brings to light all the things that are right with me too -- my perseverence, my hopes, the way I am made, my five senses to be used to meet the wonderful sounds, sights, tastes, smells and touch sensations available in the world, and my mind to use the good things of the world as they were meant to be used. There are many things right with me.

FOR TODAY: My Mind, my Heart, my Life, my Hope has been preserved, thank God. I am grateful for this miracle. I start on a new footing. I do a searching and fearless moral inventory.

"All my stories are about the action of grace on a character who is not very willing to support it." --Flannery O'Conner

W illingness is a key in Steps Four through Nine. If I am not willing at the present moment, I can pray for the willingness. Saying "yes" to life without diet remedies or excess food, we let life be a challenge, an adventure on life's terms.

FOR TODAY: I say "Hello life."

WILLING TO LOOK
FAULT-FINDING - JUDGMENT CALLS - CRITICISM   AUGUST 4

"If someone lost four pounds I thought they were the winner. Then I was off and running. What are they doing that I'm not doing? What are they using? I bet they are throwing up. I bet they don't have my metabolism. They must have more strength. Look at what they're wearing. I'll never be that size. Even if I was, I'd never look that good. Why bother. They are sitting across from me having no idea my mind is critically raging. These thoughts came around to bite me in the butt." --Anonymous

M aking judgment calls, categorizing people in all kinds of ways, and criticizing, usually brings punishing, critical thoughts that hurt me as well as others. They feed anger and resentment.

FOR TODAY: I am willing to look – just to observe – how I make judgment calls, categorize people and make criticisms in my thoughts.

"For such will be our ruin if you, in the immensity of your public abstractions, forget the private figure, or if we in the intensity of our private emotions forget the public world. Both houses will be ruined, the public and the private, the material and the spiritual, for they are inseparably connected."
--Virginia Woolf, Writer

"People sometimes say that the way things happen in the movies is unreal, but actually it's the way things happen to you in life that's unreal. The movies make emotions look so strong and real, whereas when things really do happen to you, it's like watching television—you don't feel anything."
--Andy Warhol, Artist

I have been prone to charged emotions and to numbing. When I make judgment calls, categorize or criticize, in a chilly fashion, I numb feeling, or I kick up charged emotions. I may have to avoid emotional overload, so I may feel emotions. I may have to stay away from unsafe people or set a boundary kinder to me. Being open to abuse or easily walked on is also a character defect. I may have to ask that talk about weight loss, dieting, or diet remedies be "off topic" because it brings up charged emotions.

God, Let me learn from charged emotions – what they do to me and to others. I become willing to practice restraint of tongue and pen. Charged emotions can be a quick madness or can set the ball rolling for participating in useless verbal exchanges or destructive thinking or behavior. The thrill or emotional charge of anger or resentment are not for me. I become willing to quiet any emotional disturbance.

FOR TODAY: I recall five occasions where I have been angry, scornful or critical. I watch the emotion as I recall it - rise, peak, and then let it dissipate.

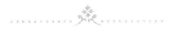

"Hate-hardened heart, O heart of iron, iron is iron til it is rust."
--Marianne Moore, Poet

Love may begin by letting go of hate, any kind of hate. The cost of abusing ourselves is too high. This character defect hurts me and others. To achieve security, acceptance, safety, belonging -- there are ways that begin by behaving with love.

God, Help me "stop think" when I abuse my mind with hate. Help me let go of anything hateful or categories with heavy charged feelings.

Seeing the world with a loving eye, I am aware of motions, movement, sounds, textures, contours, wonderful facial expressions, light, lights, colors, costumes, clothes, accoutrements, accessories in my people watching. I love the interaction of all these things. I enjoy watching people's behaviors. All this makes my reception of sensation abundant and joyful.

FOR TODAY: Traveling first class begins with me, packing love in my bag.

I n the Disney movie *1001 Dalmations,* Cruella DeVille is so vain and envious of the beauty of the puppies' coats, she wants to live in their skin. She is the height of cruelty-vanity-insanity. She is rapacious, driven by envy and want. She commits thefts, attempts murder, all because of vanity and envy. Her idea of beauty extends to wanting to live in somebody else's skin. Her singlemindedness is the height of insanity. Fortunately, the forces of goodness and the efforts of many in the community disarm her cruel actions.

I have been perplexed at envy. It has been one of my keenest resentments. It can come up so quickly. It can be so consuming, so vicious. Perhaps it comes from a primitive instinct – to want - the goods, the resources, the qualities to survive, to mate – to want.

This envy-want-fight reaction prevents me from functioning effectively. I have qualities and resources to use for my survival and adaptation. Envy takes the focus off me. An instinct that is part of the life force turns against me. Envy can destroy me.

The media has fed me on a constant diet of envy. I watch flashing images of people put forth as idols, promoted as paragons of beauty or success. Growing self-dissatisfaction emerges as I watch flashing images that have nothing to do with me personally. Advertisements about diet remedies and products feed on dissatisfaction, selling instant gratification and remedy.

God, envy can destroy my quality of living completely. It is a haunting dissatisfaction. I look at it – and the fear that my own resources are not good enough. You have created life abundant – with room for happiness, service and satisfaction.

FOR TODAY: Let me pull back from my self-denying envy when it comes up. What is really important here? I exist. I am real. Living in my own skin is one of the most sincere things I can honor. I have something of value to give. The opposite of envy is service. I reach out.

G etting honest, I examine my behavior. Where have I made excuses? An activity or obligation may have been forced on me. I may have taken on the burden, only to discover I built a resentment, or fell down, or had to bow out.

In letting go of excess food, I take a big step in letting go of social coercion. I become aware of limits. I take care of myself. I am never required to do more than I am able to do. If I need to, I say no. I respect myself.

I use the tools of Twelve Step Recovery to work through overwhelming emotions if they are preventing me from showing up. I call someone in program. I reach out to get the help I need.

I take on jobs and responsibilities where I can show up. I don't use guilt, or shaming, comparison, or coercion to force anything. I look at what I can and cannot do, for my well-being, and for the well-being of others. I don't overdo. Recognizing and living inside my limits becomes a gold standard for love, acceptance and tolerance toward myself and others.

FOR TODAY: I don't overdo or over-commit. I respect myself and play my part. I recover by remembering I am safe in the world; my contributions are good; I give up bullying against anyone, including myself. I trust.

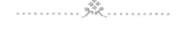

"In early abstinence and sobriety, I asked my Sponsor –'How sober am I if my bed isn't made?'" --Anonymous

"All the untidy activity continues, awful but cheerful."
--Elizabeth Bishop, Poet

Denial of the untidier aspects of myself kept me in punishing mode. Denial is a character defect too. It's called false pride and perfectionism. I see untidy emotions, habits, behaviors. I don't have to exclude them from my vision. My ears and eyes are not so sensitive.

Dear Lord, You are the Lord of all. My mind creates organization. You give me my mind. Mind is shapely. It can be inclusive. I have healthy appetites for all aspects of life, including food, affiliation, love, sexual feeling, closeness, travel, excitement, adventure, serenity, composure, learning, the unexpected, the unusual, the novel, harmony, balance.

FOR TODAY: I am willing to look. I am human. I am flesh and blood.

"I may never be satisfied with my size shape or weight."
–Anonymous

 any people think the Fourth Step is about all the wrongs we have done. It's really about waking up to ourselves.

Denial runs us. It shapes our attitudes. It takes our energy. We would rather look the other way. We would rather hide in reclusive isolation. We would rather live in fantasy. We would rather not look. In Step Four in Twelve Step Recovery, we wake up to ourselves. Whatever the conditions of our lives – about body or romance or career or family or money, we become aware. We stop running from denial. Denial means we didn't face the conditions, usually because facing that particular reality would hurt. It would be a loss of something: trust, love, family, perhaps a marriage; a friendship, or a dream. Or it would be a loss of that notion that we could demand what we wanted. We face our hurts and disappointments. They cause so much resentment and blockage.

We get out of our head. We share with God and another human being in Step Five. We become ready to accept help from another person and from our Higher Power in Step Six. We look at some of the reasons , or character defects, that have shaped our attitudes and behaviors in Step Seven. We ask for humility to deal with releasing the attitudes and misdirected thinking. We step into the light of reality. This is true awakening to conditions as they are.

FOR TODAY: I wake up to causes and conditions as they are.

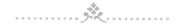

"As for health, consider yourself well."
                    --Henry David Thoreau, Writer

One reason I take a Sponsor or Spiritual Advisor is to provide balance. If I am on the depressive side, I may sink into despair bemoaning all the things I have done or the conditions that are. This is not true humility at all. This is the self-abnegation, with its gloom and doom, that drove me to the compulsive eating in the first place. Our Sponsors remind us that we have strengths. Our Sponsors remind us that despair may only be temporary, depending on the glasses we are wearing. Recovery is happening and is a lifelong process. Being abject and denying our true value is denying what our Creator has made and our God-given potentials.

Respect for our energy cycles and rhythms comes slowly with recovery. With not being on a high from mind-altering diet drugs or altered physical state, I might misread what is regular tiredness, or fatigue. Regular tiredness and fatigue happens. It does not need a mind-altering diet drug to change it. Taking power naps, time-outs to shift attention, to meditate, to calm and soothe, I recollect - I am made healthy. By re-claiming the true image of my health, TV ads, store shelves with trigger foods don't speak to me. Taking a Fourth Step I re-claim emotional and moral energy. It gives me new purpose. Healthy esteem comes from my actions. I wake up to what is right with me. Because I am living in my own skin, there is more energy and freedom to look at other things about me.

God, I accept in lovingkindness that I am a flesh and blood person. My energy cycles and rhythms are representative of human energy cycles and rhythms that have existed for millions of years. I respect and honor them. They are right and good.

FOR TODAY: I respect my body. I get adequate rest. I eat healthy and nutritious food in full amounts.

"I will always carry a small box near my heart that carries fond memories, mementoes from loved ones, small films of happy events, smiles, and warm feelings of love. It makes me very happy. It carries my sorrows too. Sometimes I take it out and look. Then I put it away and go on. When I look again – a resentment has creeped in, a fear, a harm done, another person's trouble. How did this happen? I was not meant to carry them. I have to empty them out." –Anonymous

In looking, I re-claim parts of myself that were locked off under the guise of perfectionism. I did not want to be human, a flesh and blood person with all the human emotions and character defects.

I have a disease of limited perspective. I see how limited my focus has been. It has often focused on the "poor me's", the "why me's," and all that I have been "unsatisfied with." Self-pity for what I have been given or not given carries a gloom, an anger, a resentment toward the way things "are." It excludes so many good things, possibilities, opportunities, more good things than what I could be holding in my "self-pity bag."

Continuing to look may involve a short grief, touching on other griefs, losses, or disappointments. I can never do some things again. While I can't reclaim time in my life or the fantasies of control, I can live today well and abundantly. My story helps another. I share and serve.

By looking at it all, I become a more complete and fuller person. When I unpack my "self-pity bag", then set it down to be pummelled in the rain, I can walk on, look at the trees, think about new possibilities for myself, and be grateful.

FOR TODAY: I will keep my vision clear of the fog of limited perspective. I will keep my vision open so that I may behold the wonders of all of life.

"Sex while dieting compulsively was always a problem for me. Either I was waiting until I was the size I wanted to be - to conquer. That put me in a state of denial, depriving myself of any pleasures, putting me in a generalized self-punishing mode. Or, I was in the middle of the sexual revolution, taking the liberation with the folly. " --Anonymous

aking an inventory on sex relations can reveal how our use of diet remedy substances and dieting compulsively has played into our attempts to have our desires fulfilled. An inventory can reveal where we were innocent, possibly deceived, or under self-deception. Did we rush into things out of desperation? Did experimentation turn into compulsion and addiction, much like our search for happiness from diet remedies and weight loss? What were our expectations? Were they unrealistic or excessive? Did we want more than was "possible or due us." Did self-propulsion and willful demand hurt us in our desire. Did sex relations fail through no fault of our own. Did we lack trust? Did we want control? Were we of a demanding nature? Were we in defiance rather than in reliance? The inventory can reveal humorous, humiliating, misguided, or harmful escapades. Inventory can reveal a lot about our relations with significant others and their attitudes or control issues about size shape or weight, or issues about aging and size.

FOR TODAY: My heart becomes open again in taking an inventory. I write my Fourth Step Inventory on the sex relation.

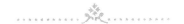

*"After I gave up diet remedies, I met a man. An angel sent me to
Room 1937 at 1 Centre Street on a temp job. There I met Jim. I
needed the job. My feet were on the ground. I needed to work. I
came into Overeaters Anonymous the same year. I was myself. I
wasn't trying to build an artificial self. I was available. I learned
love, by trusting a day at a time, and acting on my intuition
'There is something good here!' This wouldn't have been possible
if I was abusing diet remedies. I received the gift I was made
ready for."* --Anonymous

Deciding my balance with sex and love in abstinence puts me in
a more stable frame of mind. My decisions about my balance
with sex are my own and are not based on another person's views.

Having sex or not having sex does not determine my "value" or
"rating" or "grade" as a desirable attractive person. I am aware of
the difference between sex and love.

FOR TODAY: I write my goals for myself at the present moment.
I give and receive love in the world, deciding on my balance with sex
and love.

Taking the Fifth Step

"Admitted to God, to ourselves, and to another human being the exact nature of our wrongs." --Step Five, The Twelve Steps

I share my wake-up in Steps Five and Six. I no longer pretend about certain behaviors, wishes, or actions. I no longer hide under my secrets. If wrong thinking and action about dieting seemed 'normal' because others were doing it, I share about my own experience. I no longer carry the load alone about certain distressing or humiliating memories.

FOR TODAY: I am willing to let go of pride, and share with another person.

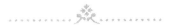

Sharing With Another Human Being

When I reach Twelve Step Recovery and stand among people who seem to understand about compulsive overeating, illness, and frustration and dissatisfaction, a great sense of belonging is experienced.

Here are real people. I am not in my head. I discover I am not alone or terminally unique.

FOR TODAY: I list five things I have never shared.

"Man was born to live with his fellow human beings. Separate him, isolate him, his character will go bad, a thousand ridiculous affects will invade his heart, extravagant thoughts will germinate in his brain, like thorns in an uncultivated land."
--Denis Diderot, French Philosopher

The man or woman who has been overeating compulsively usually feels tremendous guilt. This feeling may be based on actual wrongs done while overeating. More likely, this feeling is based on thinking about ourselves, not liking our behavior, or an internalized emotional state of doubt projected onto our body size or weight.

When others shame us, fail us, neglect or abandon us, or we are disappointed, we are ashamed of our feelings, believing there is something wrong with us. We need to remember "others are frequently wrong and often sick" as the *Twelve Steps and Twelve Traditions* says. We may respond to our feelings by hiding, shutting down, demanding more perfection of ourselves, or becoming "critic" par excellence of others. If we often retreat and don't share, feelings can become morose and despairing.

We share with another person to get some perspective. We are restored our humanity, our commonality with others. In taking Step Five, we receive understanding and forgiveness. We are able to receive and give forgiveness too. We are on our way to living our lives centered around self-respect, humanness, humility, sources of competence and service that give us pride. We are valuable human beings with something important to contribute.

For Today: When I talk to another person, I give up being frozen. I allow my emotions to exist. Perfectionism has not served me well. I allow myself to be flesh and blood.

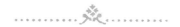

aving the obsession lifted to compulsively overeat   is a beginning on having other difficulties lifted. I move toward Higher Power's will for me. I take a break from self-propulsion. I become open to a more inclusive identity.

When I re-tell my food history with others, I find this truth-telling restores me and helps others. I begin to see how my will can align with Higher Power's will for me. My identity is no longer limited by self-will or single-minded focus on losing weight.

FOR TODAY: I abandon limited objectives. I open the door and accept direction and Higher Power. I am now ready for the Sixth Step.

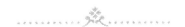

"When I was six years old I got angry and packed my Mother's suitcase and was ready to run away - until I walked down the stairs and was told by my Mother 'You can run away, but that's my suitcase. You can't take my suitcase.' Foiled. Miss Smarty Pants had been foiled. I had more growing up to do. I had to get my own suitcase. By the time I was in my 30's I had my own suitcase. I thought I was all grown up. It never occurred to me my childish impulses and need for instant gratification were all still packed in the suitcase. What an adventure to open the suitcase and get honest and show another human being what I've kept packed away over the years. Infantile fantasies, dolls, clothes. It doesn't fit anymore. I want to keep it anyway."
--Anonymous

I am free. Becoming aware sets me on a path of discovery and lifelong recovery. What an adventure to open the suitcase to get honest and show another human what has been packed away all these years.

I have learned people seek correction, guidance.

For Today: Since God can remove my obsession for eating compulsively, I let my understanding of Higher Power get bigger.

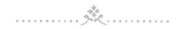

"Were entirely ready to have God remove these defects of character."
—Step Six, The Twelve Steps

I n Steps Four, Five and Six, we look at some our self-centered fears and our "unsatisfied desires." We assess what is "possible and due us." We look at "causes and conditions as they are." We get out of denial about all these things. But my character defects are so much a part of me. Giving up character defects may seem daunting.

I will be happier. This is the promise and the reality. I assume the best possible attitude on this lifelong activity.

My Creator, I am now willing that you should have all of me, good and bad. —Sixth Step Prayer, *Alcoholics Anonymous*

For Today: I make a brand new venture into open-mindnedness. I let my understanding of Higher Power get bigger.

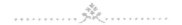

racticing trust in my Higher Power and making way for the new, I become willing to give up some of my old ideas. This emptying, this willingness to let HP provide new life, opens me up to fill up with the instinct to live and to live abundantly.

"God, Please help me set aside everything I think I know about myself, my disease, these steps, and especially You; For an open mind and a new experience with myself, my disease, these steps and especially You." –The Lay Aside Prayer

FOR TODAY: I breathe deeply, grateful for new life. I am no longer entrapped in my mind, my self-centered will, or in limited objectives. I will be guided.

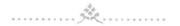

Having This Degree of Readiness   August 22

ll that Step Six asks is that we abandon our limited objectives, and move toward our Higher Power's will for us.

Having this degree of readiness keeps me on the road of recovery. In dejection and despair, in progress and movement, in bad times and in good, I get ready...

FOR TODAY: I wake-up and open up. I get ready to take action, at my own pace and my HP's pace. *"Readiness is all,"* says Shakespeare. I am engaged with my recovery in the world.

"Humbly asked Him to remove our shortcomings."
--Step Seven, The Twelve Steps

he Seventh Step begins in asking. It is not a demand. *"Humbly asked Him..."* The difference between a request and a demand is clear. This is the first place in the Twelve Steps where we ask of our Higher Power. I open myself to the reality of my Higher Power and to the ways HP speaks through others and my conscience and inner wise-mind. It is not just limited self-will.

FOR TODAY: Humbly asking is good. Arrogance, due to self-centered fear, is put aside. I get out of command mode. I place my trust in HP and others to answer what I ask, to provide.

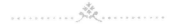

SEEING OUR DEEPER OBJECTIVES   AUGUST 24

see where I have sought to fulfill utopian material demands, or to fulfill demands about my size shape or weight. Now I see my deeper objectives. I seek to live at peace with myself and my fellows. I aim to use things to good purpose.

FOR TODAY: I ask – "Am I ever satisfied?" What am I satisfied with? I list five things I am satisfied with.

I list five unsatisfied desires. I list three unsatisfied desires about my physical body, size, shape, weight.

FOR TODAY: Am I willing to live in awareness of them rather than in denial?

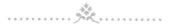

"Humility like darkness reveals the heavenly lights. The shadows of poverty and meanness gather around us, 'and lo! creation widens to our view." --Henry David Thoreau, Writer

Often it is not the fact that destroys us. It is our attitude toward the fact. Our attitude runs us. Especially when our attitude is one of controller, commander, demander, rather than humble participant or agent, we become frustrated, disappointed, and angry or resentful. When I ask God to remove my shortcomings, I can work on my attitudes about "conditions as they are." I have already opened the door to receive support in dealing with negative attitudes. Now I receive help to change my attitudes about "conditions as they are."

God, Help me take on the best possible attitude about unsatisfied desires. Help me move beyond limited objectives, toward new objectives and attitudes defined with Your help and the help of others.

FOR TODAY: I let myself be satisfied this day. The world is abundant enough for me. I include what satisfies me in my inventory. Accepting the good in love and joy, I meet obligations to myself and others in love and joy. It is enough. I am enough.

he energy I put into defense mechanisms - denial, guilt and shame, grandiosity, criticism of others, rage – railing against things as they are and my attitudes, contributes to isolation and unhappiness.

As I sort out my attitudes and the facts of my life, I get out of denial about all these things. Some of my desires – especially about size shape or weight may never be satisfied. I keep in mind deeper objectives.

Living on the basis of my humanity and humility, with the ability to forgive and be forgiven, I have deeper purpose in living. I release guilt and shame, avoid guilting or shaming others, practice kindness toward others, and give service.

I am able to move out from myself toward others and toward God.

FOR TODAY: I practice humility. I make more room in my conversations and in my decision-making, to let others in and and to let God in.

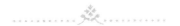

"Made a list of all persons we had harmed, and became willing to make amends to them all." --Step Eight, The Twelve Steps

I pull the names from my Fourth Step Inventory where I have looked carefully at my relationships with significant others, spouse, children, friends, siblings, parents, friends, supervisors, co-workers, and employers. Who have I harmed? Where was I to blame and who do I owe an amends to? All I have to do is make an honest list: People I am willing to make amends to now; people I am willing to make amends to later; people I will never or cannot make amends to.

FOR TODAY: All I have to do is make an honest list. I won't let fear of Step Nine keep me from being honest in Step Eight.

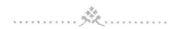

t the top of my "now" list, I put myself. I need to make amends to myself. I haven't wanted to admit the damage I was doing to my body and mind, my relationships and life possibilities. How could I have normal relationships when I wasn't thinking straight, or was thinking with grandiosity or on a buzz from mind-altering chemicals or body alterations or the denial or guilt that went with the behaviors.

God, Grant me the willingness to keep love and tolerance as my code, for myself as well as for others.

For Today: Love and tolerance is written in these amends. I do the writing.

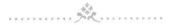

"I have been around young children and teenagers when I was using and dieting compulsively. I regret this. Children and others have observed me. " --Anonymous

o achieve health with good nutrition, there are ways that begin by behaving with love.

For Today: I want to model behaviors in front of other people that would be good for them to practice. I want to cooperate with the forces of health.

"Made direct amends to such people wherever possible, except when to do so would injure them or others."
--Step Nine, The Twelve Steps

I seek to forgive and be forgiven. I seek to repair the damage and make amends. It is important that my amends be made face-to-face, wherever possible. A face-to-face amends removes the blocks from getting right with God, with others and with myself.

Step Nine reminds me to be ever mindful not to harm others.

My Sponsor will help me in sorting out my amends list. My Sponsor will guide me in the process of taking Steps Eight and Nine, and when and where it is right to make the amends and what I am going to make an amends about. Step Nine applies to my sharing about myself at meetings or with others, as well. It reminds me not to harm myself or others in what I say, or in the time and place where I say it. I choose the right place and time for sharing. I choose health-care professionals, non-professionals, counselors, trusted friends in fellowship, and my Sponsor to share with.

"If we are painstaking about this phase of our development, we will be amazed before we are halfway through. We are going to know a new freedom and a new happiness. We will not regret the past nor wish to shut the door on it. We will comprehend the word serenity and we will know peace. No matter how far down the scale we have gone, we will see how our experience can benefit others. That feeling of uselessness and self-pity will disappear. We will lose interest in selfish things and gain interest in our fellows. Self-seeking will disappear. Our whole attitude and outlook on life will change. Fear of people and of economic insecurity will leave us. We will intuitively know how to handle situations that used to baffle us. We will realize that God is doing for us what we could not do for ourselves."
--Step Nine Promises, *Alcoholics Anonymous*, Third Edition

Having worked Steps One through Nine, I have taken the mask off. I am no longer living in denial of my realities. I have come a long way to changing my self-concept. I have exhibited courage and autonomy.

I have made an autonomous decision, deciding for myself, to let go of diet products and methods and compulsive overeating. I have decided for myself. I have challenged the myths and attitudes that would shame or coerce me to take diet substances or diet compulsively.

I have dropped pride and arrogance in the act of trusting another human being to confide in. I trust another human being and my Higher Power. I ask rather than demand. I become willing to accept guidance and direction. I take my place in community, among others. In grace and gratitude, I give up limited objectives. I am restored my humanity.

Liking my behaviors with food and in relating to others, I have less cause for resentment about anything. Comparison or envy is not necessary. I like my behaviors.

FOR TODAY: I give myself a chance by co-operating with the forces of health. I am a valuable human being. I have something important to contribute to the world. I no longer doubt myself. I have practiced courage. I continue to be courageous, to know what self-care is and to do it, to build on my identity, to work my Twelve Step program, and to experience the joy of living.

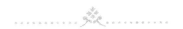

"OK God, Now what? Climbing out of my apartment I had eyes big as saucers looking skittishly at everything, wondering 'what to do now?' 'Can I take care of myself and be safe?' My first Sponsor was like an energetic grandmother. An OA beacon of light. She carried the message. I got jobs, didn't pick up or starve, and stayed out of the hospital." --Anonymous

aking care of myself means being safe when things start to happen. I am not abusing food now. I am willing to get out of my limited world.

In Steps Four through Seven I have dealt with selfishness, dishonesty, resentment, and fear. I got in touch with many things about myself. I have dealt with the past.

In Step Nine I am beginning to get the Promises. My fears are leaving me – fear of intimacy, fear of entering the world. I'm entering the world with honesty, integrity, and with my HP.

In Step Ten, when I am dealing with daily issues, and things start to crop up, I need to work my program more diligently than ever.

FOR TODAY: Higher Power is my defense against the "mental blank spot" where I may shrink back and want to use again.

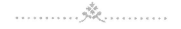

"We don't believe we exist." --Thomas Merton, Monk & Writer

"There is a vitality, a life force, an energy, a quickening that is translated through you into action, and because there is only one of you in all of time, this expression is unique. And if you block it, it will never exist through any other medium and it will be lost. The world will not have it. It is not your business to determine how good it is nor how valuable nor how it compares with other expressions. It is your business to keep it yours clearly and directly, to keep the channel open. You do not even have to believe in yourself or your work. You have to keep yourself open and aware to the urges that motivate you. Keep the channel open." --Martha Graham, Dancer

ou are supposed to exist in your current form. The whole universe confirms you - you are a one-time unique person. You do exist.

FOR TODAY: I believe I exist.

"There's a period in life when we swallow a knowledge of ourselves and it becomes either good or sour inside."
                    --Pearl Bailey, Singer

"Charts and formulas given out by the diet program companies showed how many calories and how many pounds I would lose in what time." –Anonymous

I will be with myself much longer than charts and formulas a diet program company may offer me. I value my unique physiology, biology, talents, temperament, emotional acre, and abilities, the individual I am.

FOR TODAY: Taking care of myself begins with valuing myself.

"Integrity is the acceptance of one's one and only life cycle and the people who have become significant to it... It is a sense of comradeship with men and women of distant times and of different pursuits who have created orders and objects and sayings conveying human dignity and love... The lack or loss of this accrued ego integration is signified by disgust and by despair."
          --Erik Erikson, Psychologist & Writer

"Can someone have integrity taking diet drugs and diet remedies? Sure. The same way someone can have integrity who uses alcohol. Integrity has something to do with integral, being held together. The diet drugs just tore me apart. At first subtly then very dramatically." –Anonymous

When I live authentically, respecting my physiology, my biology, my talents, my limits, and the positive efforts I make to develop myself, I am nourished by my integrity and self-respect. I do not want another life. I accept the life I have. I am freed from disdain and scorn.

Sometimes I am in despair – but my despair is not a permanent condition.

For Today: I take responsibility and choose to love the real and to love life.

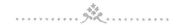

"The world is my storehouse. I can run. Or I can enter into some kind of relationship with people. It's a dance I don't know. I don't have all the steps. The dance is always new. There are stops and starts." –Anonymous

"Making my concept of my Higher Power bigger allows me to enter the world. It is a real world, a world full of real people and possibilities for real satisfactions." –Anonymous

"Today in my inventory, I included, welcomly receiving a hug from a favored co-worker, Mike. I was sitting in my desk chair, with a warm red cashmere sweater and he touches my hair. Then I said - thank you, I have something for you too. I have news for you about when the raises will be in our checks...' It was a real hug of love and I welcomed it. I am not in fantasy head but in real head. I also am glad for the friendly co-worker." --Anonymous

FOR TODAY: I can go beyond my comfort level and still be safe.

I am no longer in the problem. I am in the solution. I am taking care of myself with healthy food in healthy amounts. I am working my program diligently. I am not numb. I am alive. Gratitude lists, Top 10 Happy Memory Lists, Happy Times with a Particular Person, shift perspective and remind me that any pain, un-acceptance or aversion to any moment is not the total picture. HP will change my perception of the present moment. My HP gives me the presence of mind to practice active patience. An answer and an intuition will come.

God, Direct my thinking to how you would have me be. I pray for release from resentment and anger, and lashful tongues. I pray for the sick and suffering.

FOR TODAY: I am alive.

When things start to happen, being a witness to my life requires clear thinking. I practice clear thinking about my emotions, emotional triggers, internal verbal landscape, thoughts, feelings, judgments, and sensations. I learn to identify these components. I practice awareness, mindfulness, and radical acceptance without judgment.

"You don't just think. You think about something."
--Sherman Paul, Writer

I practice clear thinking - about what is going on, what I am feeling, then about what is the work at hand. Very often I have not known what I was feeling. Awareness brings me in touch with what I need to do, based on where I am emotionally, spiritually, physically, financially. It tells me what my "habitat" is, my inner landscape and the conditions and people surrounding me. What do I need to do to live manageably today? What do I need to do to paddle my own canoe so it doesn't shear on the rocks, so it moves with the waters and respects the conditions and other things that are there?

How many colors and hues of happiness, joy, satisfaction, pleasure, gratification, enjoyment are there? Or shades of sadness, unhappiness, disappointment or irritability?

Let me observe my present emotional state.

I practice clear thinking to identify and solve a problem. I practice clear thinking by "putting on my thinking cap" to do work, to start a project, to create a project, to do an assignment, or to use my "skills at learning", to learn something and then to address creating something out of it.

FOR TODAY: I take care of myself by practicing clear thinking.

"Shutting down before I start traps me. When I went to a chorus rehearsal for the first time, I almost left 5 minutes before the rehearsal began. I sat through the feelings and told myself 'I am safe. I am safe.' I love it now." –Anonymous

With unavoidable or unpredictable triggers that remind me of something stressful, shopping for clothes or meeting new people, I can become trapped in an old way of thinking or an old fear. I can become paralyzed, or lash out, or engage in self-destructive behavior acting out with compulsive dieting or food.

Today I don't further "emotion brain." I don't need to react ineffectively – get distressed, blame someone else or myself, aggrandize, dramatize, or be overly fearful. I can acknowledge the situation and stop trying to fight the moment.

FOR TODAY: I am in the present. I use all my faculties.

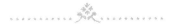

I have to know what I am feeling and be in contact with my Higher Power in order to stay spiritually fit. This is where I discuss with my Sponsor or another trusted person about incidents that bother me. I learn more about my part. I see the satisfactions of new behavior, entering the world, trying new behaviors, trusting a Power greater than myself, my Higher Power, to help me be safe and effective.

Let me be a witness to my life. Let me observe my rational self and emotional self, and the intersecting point, where my recovered mind sees both and takes action. Let me act on a higher plane, about anger, understanding, kindness and ethics.

FOR TODAY: I "Practice Courage" in staying in the world, not discounting myself, not hiding. I move toward my good, in order to live fully, to serve, and to help others.

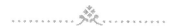

"We are all instruments endowed with feeling and memory. Our senses are so many strings that are struck by surrounding objects and that also frequently strike themselves."
                    --Denis Diderot, Philosopher & Writer

How often I forget how green the grass is -- the colors and shapes of the trees -- all that I have -- my wonderful senses operating all the time. Being conscious upfront brings me in touch with -- my breathing, my sensations of smell, vision, hearing.

My sensations can bring me a lot. I can self-soothe - using my breathing, my sense of smell, my sense of vision, my sense of hearing. I may have an aversion to being where I am – the moment will change if I give time time. Soothing by going toward all that is going on with my sensations and perceptions, soothes charged emotions. It brings me into safe place emotionally.

By enlarging my Higher Power, daily, I take stock of my surroundings. Am I comfortable within myself? Do I give myself the cleanliness, warmth and caring I need? Do I rest and relax? These physical senses delight me.

Do I need to reduce the clashing of surrounding sensations, ideas, images, thoughts, overload on my senses?

FOR TODAY: My wonderful five senses and the sensations of the present reality bring me pleasure. I find pleasure in the changing moment -- light, sights, colors, sounds, contours, textures, shapes -- the fullness of life.

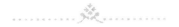

"Everything you need you already have. You are complete right now, you are a whole, total person, not an apprentice person on the way to someplace else. Your completeness must be understood by you and experienced in your thoughts as your own personal identity....There are no short cuts to anywhere worth going."
--Beverly Sills, Opera Singer & Opera Director

"I like myself much better now that I am not overeating. Every day there is energy for other activities. Working with others, I'm organizing a boat ride for people in my program."
--Anonymous

When I align my will with complete acceptance of reality, the whole world stands behind me. In denial I am alone. When I deny my existence, my self-worth, I am not in alignment with reality. I do not see the good others see. Self-centered pride focuses my energies on denying my existence.

The creative effort focuses my energies on going forward with talents, confidence, cheerfulness in spite of the shadows defining the contours of the light.

"If my rough hammer in hard stone can form,
A human semblance, one and then another,
Set moving by the agent who is holder,
Watcher and guide, its course is not its own."
--Michelangelo, Sculptor & Poet

The man who could take a shape out of stone must have had faith in the form there that was to be found. We need to have faith in our own forms.

For Today: All that I have I honor. I take a breath. I listen to the various sounds around me, the space between sounds. Trusting my Higher Power with me brings me comfort and confidence.

"Close your eyes and get quiet for a minute, until the chatter starts up. Then isolate one of the voices and imagine the person speaking as a mouse. Pick it up by the tail and drop it into a mason jar. Then isolate another voice, pick it up by the tail, drop it in the jar. And so on. Drop in any high-maintenance parental units, drop in any contractors, lawyers, colleagues, children, anyone who is whining in your head. Then put the lid on, and watch all these mouse people clawing at the glass, jabbering away, trying to make you feel like shit because you won't do what they want....Then imagine that there is a volume control button on the bottle. Turn it all the way up for a minute...Then turn it all the way down and watch the frantic mice lunge at the glass trying to get to you. Leave it down and get back to your shitty first draft."

--Anne Lamott, Writer

The challenge of living each day well starts with clearing the mind and setting to live in truth and integrity. That means clearing my head of food talk, either romancing the food or criticizing myself, and going forth with actual plans for meals.

When I observe overwhelming emotions and visualize safe-place again, I recover a sense of well-being. The need to combat the attack voices and the voices of self-loathing by using diet remedies like armors and shields and masks goes away. There is no cause. Things are right.

People only have as much power as I give them. Right sizing other people is important. I would not be here if millions of years of "right fit" did not cooperate to bring me here. With the right elements and combination of air, water, light, from my ancestor survivors, I was born to survive and prosper.

FOR TODAY: I watch my banshees, phantoms, and monsters take a hike. Before I am overwhelmed with anything painful, I get my pleasure centers working. Humor perhaps? Visualizing a clever way to banish the bears?

"Awareness is learning to keep yourself company."
                    --Geneen Roth, Writer

"'Don't dial pain.' That's what a trusted friend, like a big sister in my Overeaters Anonymous program, told me. What good advice for being a good friend!" –Anonymous

I am in a better position to be good company to myself after doing my Fourth Step Inventory. All the moths are out of the closet.

I don't dial pain.

I can keep myself in good company. With other people, I can walk away. I can come back on my terms.

To accept being imperfectly un-comparably human, I live in existing integrity and don't dial despair. That's what being good company means to me. I dance with the plums in the refrigerator. I run them under the water.

FOR TODAY: What is good company to me? I define it. I put it into motion. Good company gives me confidence to enjoy the world. It assures me I can take care of myself.

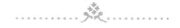

"The great artist sees his objects (and this is true whether they are sad, absurd, repulsive or even evil) in a light of justice and mercy. The direction of attention is, contrary to nature, outward, away from self which reduces all to a false unity, towards the great surprising variety of the world, and the ability so to direct attention is love." --Sissela Bok, Writer

"It's so not about me. When I work with others in 12 Step Recovery, it's about them." --Anonymous

Generosity of spirit, seeing things and people in the light of justice and mercy, means that I recognize the artistry that exists beyond my tastes. There is more than I know, since I know only a very few things and a very few people really well.

I am willing to claim my humanity. I am willing to work with others to show them that there is a way to their humanity that doesn't involve using or cover-ups or demands on them to change body size.

FOR TODAY: I am part of life. Life is hard enough and confusing. There are demands on everyone. Love and tolerance are my code.

"When Jesus was asked about beauty, he pointed to nature, to the lilies of the field. Behold them, he said, and behold is a special word: it means to look upon something amazing or unexpected...Jesus is saying that every moment you are freely given the opportunity to see through a different pair of glasses....Jesus is saying that we have much to learn from them about giving up striving. He's not saying that in a "Get over it" way, as your mother or last, horrible husband did. Instead, he's heartbroken, as when you know an anorexic girl who's starving to death, as if in some kind of demonic possession. He's saying that we could be aware of, filled with, and saved by the presence of holy beauty, rather than worship golden calves." --Anne Lamott, Writer

"Blessed are they which do hunger and thirst after righteousness: for they shall be filled." -- *Bible:* New Testament - Matthew 5:6

My thirst is noble. Thirst for the way to take care of my true self is noble. I will be loved for myself - not only when I am good for my goodness, when I cannot be expected to be good all the time, not only when my body is young or unblemished, not only when my body is a certain size, shape or weight. Many people love me this way.

Whatever my spiritual or religious practice, it is revolutionary to say - I have the ability to take care of myself, to be safe and healthy, and I can recognize this way for me, and thirst for it, and be free and supported in the way I have chosen.

For Today: I can be fulfilled. I have appreciation for the life I have been given and the life that has been preserved.

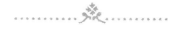

"Why should we all dress after the same fashion? The frost never paints my windows twice alike."
          --Lydia Maria Child, Abolitionist, Women's Rights Activist

"Every single one of us at birth is given an emotional acre all our own." -- Anne Lamott, Writer

"If I want tolerance, I have to give it too." –Anonymous

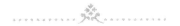he Twelve Step programs encourage listening, and no cross-talk at meetings. By listening to others, I learn how unique and different from one another, yet similar, people really are. I gain strength. I am supported in the personal ways I have chosen to nourish my health, sanity, and spiritual growth.

I don't have to debate, give advice, be critical or judge. Likewise, I am safe. I give tolerance.

FOR TODAY: I take care of myself by abstaining from compulsive eating. This is what I need.

"The worst part of success is to try to find someone who is happy for you." --Bette Midler, Singer-Dancer-Actress

O thers may not give me attention or the appreciation I crave because of their self-enhancement needs or self-centeredness. That doesn't mean my self-worth or accomplishment is zero. My approval and accomplishment mean a great deal to me.

"I perform on Broadway. My family hasn't come to see me. Yes, it hurts. I let go. I release them. I go on in joy. I am certain of my talents. Respect is there for me. Fellowship too from friends and my talent community." --Anonymous

"I match up newcomers with Sponsors at a meeting with 400 people." --Anonymous

"I got 457 votes in my Union Local election from people I work with. They know who I am and like me and voted for me. This is awesome to me. It is such affirmation." --Anonymous

Being happy for myself – I respect and enjoy my accomplishments.

I travel with myself 24/7. It is quiet happiness to share and to see the light in men and women's faces who have given up problems with the help of their individual Higher Powers, who accomplish and enjoy their satisfactions.

Lord, today I pray for continued health and well-being. I pray to serve the health and well-being of others.

FOR TODAY: I choose happiness.

We are always being told about desire. We are being prompted to fill our desire. By seeing my "unsatisfied desires," in my Fourth Step work, and evaluating whether they are "possible or due me", or worthy, I empty out some unfulfilled desires that keep me chasing, and make room to enjoy real pleasures.

My energies are released to focus on the pleasures that exist and can exist for me.

Healthy legs walking briskly, a good cup of coffee, clean clothes, pets, a few coins to spend, people watching, beautiful relationships, baubles-bangles-beads, lovely people, sunshine on my face -- whatever gives me real obtainable pleasure, I take. I put some pleasurable activities in my day.

Giving love gives me pleasure. It affirms I have something of value to contribute. It is the gift I give that asks no reward. A perfect smile, a kind word. Paying attention to someone. Praising, seeing the good. Seeing the beauties in others.

FOR TODAY: Staying spiritually fit means taking pleasures in the real world daily.

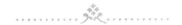

aying 'I Want' and 'I Need' is an excellent practice for clarifying who I am.

I may have been numb, or denied that I have needs. Or I may have felt that my needs were so great that they could not be met. I may have felt, "why bother asking?" I may have felt, "why identify what I want and need?" I may have de-selfed. I only took care of other people, not myself.

I may have been in relationships with people who cannot or will not be available to meet my needs. I may have asked and the answer was "no." I may have asked the wrong source. I may need to ask another source. Or, I may have been abundantly and pleasantly surprised by people who read my emotional needs and met them in wonderful ways. I will be pleased again as people meet my wants and needs.

I say "I want and I need" to things I am able to provide for myself. I also say "I want and I need" to things I want from other people.

God, Help me have the right attitude in asking. No single individual is able to provide for my needs and wants. God, You are my Source. It is up to me to do my thinking. You will lead me to right sources.

Help me ask the appropriate source, where they are able and willing to provide. I am not a burden to people I ask. If a person says "no," let me accept their answer. I can process whatever emotion comes with the answer and move on with emotional sobriety. I continue to recognize the validity of my wanting or needing. Your world is abundant. There are abundant resources.

Let my contracts and agreements be clear. Let me be clear if I am making a work request where I will pay a fair fee in exchange for work I need done. Let me use my talents and abilities to pay money for work I need from others. Employing others allows them to use their talents, abilities and enthusiasms. Let me give a fair wage to others for their work.

"Hiring people on a task or per hour basis feels right. Instead of feeling self-pity, I reach out. Others are there to help! A handyman makes small repairs. A personal assistant helps me get started over coffee for the day and does work for my small business. A neighbor's son does errands." --Anonymous

At night, when I do my daily Inventory and prepare for tomorrow, I clarify my thinking. I include this question in my meditation: "What do I want and need?" Now this question is clearly in front of me. It helps me take care of myself. What do I want and need to do? For the next day? What do I want to do for the near future and longer term future? I make specific realistic attainable plans.

FOR TODAY: I nourish my needs for affiliation, security, stability, and the material and spiritual goods of this world. Saying "I want and I need" is different from living on the basis of vague "unsatisfied demands." I say "yes, I want and I need" to things that are right, to what I want for myself and others. I say "yes" to work that is right for me. I make a commitment for goals, job, work, creative projects, friendships, family, and relationships. It is a joy.

"There goes another one. A radio ad for a weight loss product.
There goes another one. A TV ad for a weight loss product."
                  –Anonymous

wareness of the messages I receive around me, and the messages I give myself, enables me to see the input in my life. Messages are received all the time – from movies, TV, Internet advertising, text and pictures on product advertising and what the people in my life communicate to me about their thoughts about me and about their life and values.

Awareness enables me to test the truth of messages or their quality of life. In observing, I can see impersonal advertising messages in my environment that urge me to eat or diet, to compare or discount, to correct or to change. Are the messages hostile or friendly? Do they refer to me by name? Do they know me?

Then by being conscious I can turn to my Higher Power and make decisions and choices about what I want to accept, what is true, what is valuable to me and how, or what I like and want or don't like or don't want. It is important for me to observe my surrounding environment. Most media messages give alarm messages. I have the ability to take care of myself. I can keep my personal daily environment safe. I need to remember this.

"There is a moment in 'The Heiress' when Olivia de Havilland realizes Montgomery Clift loves her and her father has duped her into believing she is unattractive and unlovable and unworthy all these years. It is a startling moment. To me, it is the best moment in the whole movie. She wakes up. She is no longer a prisoner of someone who defines her negatively. She is a beautiful woman. She is a free woman." –Anonymous

FOR TODAY: I have a sense of myself. I detach from erroneous messages.

"Don't dial pain." –Anonymous

"For as we brutalize our sensitivities, we narrow the possibilities of serving with our own spiritual and mental health."
                    –Kenneth O. Jones, Minister & Writer

Choosing to be around safe people is possible. I have to get to know them. Being sensitive to my own emotional triggers, I learn if they are going to push my buttons? I choose not to brutalize my sensitivities by being around the sordid or the mean.

Choosing to go to safe places is possible. I can go to places where I will not be challenged for my thoughts and feelings. Likewise, I don't challenge others for their thoughts and feelings. It is safe for each of us.

I go to safe hip places where the focus is not on body size, shape, or weight but another focus. An environment group, civic betterment group, playwriting or writing group, singing group for enjoyment and purpose are places where I can practice what I have learned about taking care of myself and get to know people.

FOR TODAY: It's ok for me to make choices that work. I don't have to be open for abuse or upset. Opening and closing my receptors, my eyes, my ears, my time, I can be around safe people and create safer places for myself.

H ow much time do I want to spend on the phone with someone? I learn to say "I have to jump now...". I learn to end conversations.

The safe boundary I create is for the other person too. Letting others compulse about an issue does them a disservice. I quiet the disturbance.

"Every so often someone wants a debate in the wrong place like at work. My values are my own. When someone wants to get into an intense conversation about finances, religion, sex, family, food and diet, I change the subject, or say my thoughts are personal, or even, if I'm particularly vulnerable, I have to go now. It's not perfect. I let people know what I want them to know about me and my values when I feel safe and safe about them."

--Anonymous

In recovery, by entering the world, we are bound to meet people who are walking advertisements. They advertise what they do and promote it. Diets, exercise techniques. We don't have to buy in. We have the ability to decide for ourselves. We are allowed to make mistakes.

FOR TODAY: This adventure called life calls on me to use my navigating abilities - to get to the right places and to stop at the right resting spots, and to exercise my in-born abilities to take care of myself. I do that the best ways I can. I am in tune with myself, what feels right. If it doesn't feel right, I do the best I can to change it - to keep on living and enjoying life.

veryone has to deal with others. As a recovering compulsive overeater, it is important I don't "de-self". I need to hold on to my integrity, not be invisible, stay in the field, in the arena, as this person. I cannot let myself be haunted by distress or chased into hiding or hunted by intimidation. I learn effective ways to take care of myself. A shy person may still exist inside me – but I enter the world as I am without terror. I have ways to deal.

Being powerless over other people's behaviors means I do not do "their" behaving. I do not have ability to control other people as a puppet on a string or remotely control them. Other people do their own behaving. If other people hit verbally, or physically, use sordid or mean language, it is their behavior. If they are sweet or kind, it is their behavior. Everyone has their own Higher Power.

My reaction or response to other people's behavior is my responsibility. I have many choices.

I am available to myself. I focus on my behavior. I have choices.

FOR TODAY: I don't live in fear.

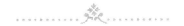

"My best friend in OA always says 'Ask five people.' I've started doing that now, turning any bafflement, distress, or general 'not knowing' into a party of opinions. It's not that I take advice easily. I'm a proud woman. I break isolation. I start to involve other people in my life." –Anonymous

"'This video game is upsetting me. I can't win. What do I do? Do I send it back? My cousin gave it to me.' I got different opinions from several people. The takes I liked the best were 'You have a right to enjoy your life. Don't let anything upset you that causes too much pressure,' from the young friend. 'Don't waste your energy. It's wasted energy on that,' from a co-worker I like. They were the best takes for me. They resonated best."
                                        --Anonymous

It's surprising. Other people have usually been there in some way and have an experience with something I'm wondering about. Letting others in, I ask. It's a way of letting go of isolation, pride, grandiosity. I get relatedness. They know more about me by what I ask. I know more about them by what they say.

For Today: I let others in.

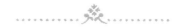

aking care of myself involves using some of those rules I learned as a child: play fair.

I watch. I wear the hat of a parent and self parent. I don't let my children play with children who run with scissors or hit. I need to stay away from adults who do the same thing. Fearing adults who run with scissors can keep me in compulsive dieting or overeating. "You beat me. I'll beat you. I'll be the best beater. I'll get so good, so thin, so perfect, you can't attack me."

I remember, I can't control the unexpected. I can't control other people's behavior. It is their nature and not something about me. I remember, chances are what they are doing to me, they are doing to ten other people. *"Finally, we begin to see that all people, including ourselves, are to some extent emotionally ill as well as frequently wrong,"* it says in *The Twelve Steps and Twelve Traditions.*

When I stay off the court and don't entertain attack and counter-attack games, it is better for everyone. Sometimes leaving a situation is the only thing I can do. I vote with my feet. Emotional sobriety is important.

FOR TODAY: Taking care of myself involves using some of those rules I learned as a child for playing fair.

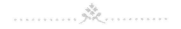

"My co-worker slapped his hand down on the desk, said something nasty, and stomped away! It was scarry, like he was hitting me. He got angry and was refusing to train me. I pulled a book down from my shelf 'Success With the Gentle Art of Verbal Self-Defense' by Suzette Elgin. It said 'Don't take the bait. Recognize you are under attack. Modulate an attack with something in leveler voice, like 'No comment' or 'I see your feeling'. Formulate a complaint.' I formulated a complaint and took it to my Supervisor. We all met. I read my complaint. 'When you get angry and refuse to train me, you are preventing me from doing my job.' I felt safer. Being threatened in the workplace can affect my showing up. I need to work. When my co-worker retired we hugged." –Anonymous

"Verbal violence is next to physical violence."--Suzette Elgin, Writer

Inflections that emphasize certain words, and phrases like "Even you...", or "You never..." or "You always...", or "If you really..." clue us in to verbal violence. We can observe just how much verbal violence is in our daily surroundings. I don't internalize the language patterns of verbal abuse. We can be prepared and feel safer as we live in the world. We can learn not to take the bait, to de-escalate the attack by using leveler voice, and formulate a complaint when ready.

FOR TODAY: If there is verbal violence, I know how to deal with it.

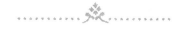

"A man cornered me in the elevator and said, 'My wife is like you. She carries all her weight around her hips like you.' I said, 'Yes. I'm not big other places.' Uncomfortable, caught off guard, I got off at my elevator stop. It bothered me, his talking about my body and feeling trapped. I sent him an email. 'That was unprofessional of you to talk about my body, when you said... Please don't behave unprofessionally again. If you do, I will have to report it to my Director, Personnel and EEO.'" –Anonymous

"Body molesting through talk makes me feel naked and exposed."
--Anonymous

arassment is harassment. Even with a smile on its face or as a left-handed compliment, harassment is intended to disturb or upset. Harassment refers to a wide spectrum of offensive behaviour. When the term is used in a legal sense, it refers to behaviors which are found threatening or disturbing.

In the experience of harassment, someone has violated my boundaries, has offended me. I have not violated their boundaries. I have no reason for any guilt or shame. I do not need to be a victim. Recognition translates into right action if harassment happens.

I say - 'I don't like it. I want you to stop it. If you don't stop it, or do it again, I will take further action.'

FOR TODAY: I do not need to be uncomfortable in the workplace. I have the right to work today.

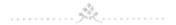

ow that I am recovering, I am willing to challenge unuseful thoughts.

I will intuitively know what to do using all my faculties to guide me in my best good, practicing active patience, and challenging unuseful thoughts.

God, I pray for You to help me challenge unuseful thoughts.

I take out the garbage when I vent safely the aggravations of the day, wind down safely, and challenge unuseful thoughts, thoughts that would do no purposeful good.   I will not fear what does not exist.   I will not spin dramas that are more smoke than warmth from a working fire.

FOR TODAY: I will evaluate what is useful to specific manageable attainable realistic goals. What are my priorities today? What recent unuseful thoughts do I need to challenge?

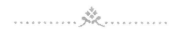

"I have relied on fear instincts. Using diet drugs and eating compulsively was a way of combating fear and distracting me from facing life problems. Real fear based on a real threat needs to be addressed." --Anonymous

"Fear is an emotion indispensable for survival."
                    --Hannah Arendt, Writer

annah Arendt's quote comes from her writings on the personal and political apathy, the banality of evil, that let people be hounded, persecuted, driven into hiding, deprived of work, and murdered in Germany, the Netherlands, Austria, Poland, Hungary and France in the 1930's and 1940's. She talks about the fear of those who participated and stood by because they feared for their survival.

Many people fear being on the wrong side of the 'diet now' and 'thin is well' drumbeat.

Am I apathetic? Have I been fearful and chased into punishing compulsive dieting? Have I chased others into it or scorned people?

Being a Stand-Up Person and practicing courage is a good practice. It makes me stronger in the world – more able to contribute.

FOR TODAY: I will assess carefully.

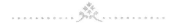

"Stability is good. It is good waking up in the morning knowing what my body will feel like. It is good knowing what my family can expect of my behavior. I plan what I am going to eat for the day."
                    --Anonymous

ear God, Thank you for Your guidance in helping me set my goals for today. Thank you for prompting me to ask about my purposes. I take an action with purpose. Thank you for giving me trusted others to talk to, including my Sponsor and my trusted friends.

What can I do today to make my emotions, my finances, my relationships, my job relationships and work activity more stable?

To honor God's will, I plan my food. I make sure that the right food in the right amounts is available to me.

FOR TODAY: What actions today will make my life manageable.

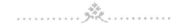

"Wrap us in the web of mutual caring and concern. Keep us from coldness of heart toward each other."
                                    –Kenneth O. Jones, Writer & Minister

"We don't see things as they are, we see them as we are."
                                    --Anais Nin, Writer

W e will spend all of our lives with ourselves. Our opinion of ourselves matters. Being kind to ourselves matters. Being kind to ourselves is a conscious awareness and practice vital for creating a safe world and sticking up for kindness to others.

My self-care will have a ripple effect. It will contribute to a model of behavior that doesn't chase after idolatries, pursuits that will not fill me, or others, or the useless or unnecessary. Enjoyment of the essential comes naturally to me.

"Things base and vile, holding no quantity,
Love can transpose to form and dignity.
Love looks not with the eyes, but with the mind,
And therefore is winged Cupid painted blind."
--William Shakespeare, *A Midsummer Night's Dream*

Breathing together with others, especially with others in Twelve Step Recovery, I get peace and comfort. I am one among many, and unique. My search for sundry ordinary answers is elevated. I get to begin with the simplest of questions about things I don't know how to do. I get to ask questions about how to take care of myself and best serve others.

FOR TODAY: I relax. I don't have to do it alone. I can take care of myself. An answer and an intuition will come.

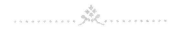

"Identity formation begins where the usefulness of identification ends." –Erik Erikson, Psychologist & Writer

Usually identity formation begins for a girl or a boy when they recognize they are separate from their oneness identification with their Mother. They begin a unique unfolding that shows them their individual feelings, capabilities, limits, and abilities.

Likewise, I build on identity when I separate from a mirror that says "lose weight" any way possible. I see myself as I am, as myself. I recognize boundaries - where I begin and where I end. I recognize limits - what I can do and what I cannot do. I separate from unuseful identification with media images. I see abilities and enthusiasms. I build on abilities and enthusiasms with the new energy that is released.

FOR TODAY: While I will always be recovering, and someone who has abused diet products and methods and food, today I am recovered. I have a daily reprieve. I am no longer a member of the debating society.

"When I was a child..." --Bible, 1 Corinthians 13:11

I am willing to build on a solid foundation and to build on identity. To do this, I keep my awareness of my new knowledge about myself and my awakening in front of me. I continue to take personal inventory. I take Step Ten. I take spot-check inventories. I cease fighting anything or anybody. I take further action. In prayer and meditation, I ask for daily guidance. I use all my mental faculties. My thought life is placed on a higher plane. I place my life on a higher plane of living.

"I am willing to grow along spiritual lines. I have learned about my emotions and instincts. I have learned how much stress I can carry without short-changing those I'm responsible to. This knowledge is invaluable to me." --Anonymous

"Becoming" as psychologists from Abraham Maslow and others say, is an arduous process. It involves creativity. It involves recognizing the raw materials of creation, and how we want to live creatively and become...

May I proceed in confidence. I work with my knowledge about self, my abilities, and my potentials for growth. God gives me direction. It takes perseverence, tenacity, courage, and creativity.

For Today: I tap into the creative Universe.

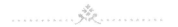

"Continued to take personal inventory, and when we were wrong promptly admitted it." --Step Ten, The Twelve Steps.

We continue to watch for selfishness, dishonesty, resentment and fear. When these crop up, we ask God to remove them. This line of *The AA Big Book* says "when these crop up," NOT "if they crop up." Our inventory-taking is a life-long activity. Step Ten is to be taken throughout the day, as these things crop up. *"We discuss them with someone immediately."*

May I continue to take personal inventory and set right any new mistakes as I go along. I vigorously commenced this way of living as I cleaned up the past.

FOR TODAY: I take spot-check inventories as I go along.

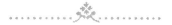

CEASING TO FIGHT ANYBODY OR ANYTHING   OCTOBER 5

The early founders of Alcoholics Anonymous learned they could no longer enter into the beer or wine versus hard liquor debate. Likewise, I have resigned from the debating society. I don't enter into any debate about this trigger food versus that. By this time sanity has returned. If tempted by trigger foods, I recoil from them. I am neither cocky nor am I afraid.

My living problems also cease to be a fight. I ask whether acceptance or change is required. Approaching living with the right heart is right.

FOR TODAY: May I remember that fight or flight is an instinctive response to fear. Fight or flight isn't the only response. May I stop reactions that are not effective, and draw on the experience, strength and hope of others in Twelve Step Recovery to help.

BUILDING ON IDENTITY

"Sought through prayer and meditation to improve our conscious contact with God." --Step Eleven, The Twelve Steps"

"God has given you a chance to make a spirit within yourself. By prayer I don't mean shouting and mumbling and wallowing like a hog in religious sentiment. Prayer is only another name for good clean direct thinking. When you pray think. Think well what you are saying. Make your thoughts on things that are solid. That way your prayer will have strength. That strength will become part of you, body, mind and spirit." --Walter Pidgeon (*Mr. Griffith from 'How Green Was My Valley' - John Ford*)

o some extent I have become God-conscious. But I go further and that means more action. Step Eleven suggests in prayer and meditation --

I ask that I be shown what my next step for the day is to be.
I ask to be given what I need to take care of problems.
I ask for freedom from self-will.
I make requests that are not for myself alone, for selfish ends.
I ask for freedom from the danger of excitement, fear,
anger, worry, self-pity, or foolish decisions.

FOR TODAY: I practice courage by staying in the world. I will not discount myself. I will not hide. I seek guidance from my Higher Power as I go. I move toward my highest good. I serve and help others.

"I thought I was finished... with the weight battle. I was done. I'd conquered it. I was so sure, I was even cocky. I had the nerve to say to friends who were struggling, 'All you have to do is work out harder and eat less!'" --Oprah Winfrey, Media Producer & Actress

My life is a journey. I live it one day at a time. New insights are gained all the time. Part of my Tenth Step Inventory each day will include - where was I unkind? Where was I demanding? Where was my acceptance not real? Where did I only want to deal with the gifted child, in Alice Miller's term in *The Drama of the Gifted Child* - myself - for her gifts, her goodness, her body size shape or weight?

My Eleventh Step morning meditation will ask. 'Will love and tolerance be my code today?' I accept acceptance. God only asks of me to do the best I can.

FOR TODAY: I can decide what is my path for today. By working to stay spiritually fit, I am granted a daily reprieve from compulsive overeating. I continue my journey. I can only work my program, not somebody else's, one day at a time.

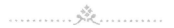

"The significant problems we face cannot be solved at the same level of thinking we were at when we created them."
                    --Albert Einstein, Scientist

FOR TODAY: Using all my faculties, takes my thinking to a higher plane. I have a new design for living.

"The human mind possesses a special advantage over the brain: for once it has created impressive symbols and has stored significant memories, it can transfer its characteristic activities to materials like to stone and paper that outlast the original brain's brief life-span. When the organism dies, the brain dies, too, with all its lifetime accumulations. But the mind reproduces itself by transmitting its symbols to other intermediaries, human and mechanical, than the particular brain that first assembled them." --Lewis Mumford, Writer

his is a book of meditations. The act of meditating is an active act. I learn from meditating on the writings of others, what they have thought and shared. I am willing to go to my Higher Power to help me discern what is valuable to me.

FOR TODAY: Upon awakening, I meditate.   Today I will learn something useful.

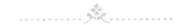

"Life is a good teacher, though an expensive one."
--Author Unknown

"And the green grass grows all around all around. And the green grass grows all around." --American Folk Song

There are margins for error. They are wider than we think, given our perfectionism. Error may be costly. Yet the green grass keeps growing. The wheat fields will yield a crop. My loved ones and neighbors, we will all have our share. We need to have vision.

My education continues.

Life teachers -- parents, good friends, children in my presence, co-workers, teachers, those people I identify as my personal spirit guides -- give me lessons to guide me. I observe, listen, learn and am glad of it.

"We must remain teachable."
--*Alcoholics Anonymous*, Third Edition

Building on my identity comes. I let go of self-will and open up to receive from life teachers. The loving arms of God are wide.

FOR TODAY: Each step I take in confidence. I bring experience, wisdom and vision along.

"We will intuitively know how to handle things which used to baffle us." Alcoholics Anonymous, Third Edition

"If you feel your value lies in being merely decorative, I fear that you someday might find yourself believing that's all that you really are. Time erodes all such beauty. But what cannot diminish is the wonderful workings of your mind, your humor, your kindness, and your moral courage."
  --Susan Sarandon *(Marmee from 'Little Women'- Jane Austen)*

I have an "Openness" to the new, now that I am living on new principles. This awareness goes beyond "Education" from parents, teachers, or school. It goes beyond "Smarts." It goes beyond "Looks."

FOR TODAY: My Higher Power gives me active patience, calm, guidance in opening myself to the new -- body, mind & spirit.

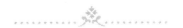

"It took me a long painful time to move beyond dollhouse thinking - wanting a ready-made husband, a ready-made house, ready-made children. " --Anonymous

uthentic dreams and daydreams, based on an awakening to the Great Reality spurs us on. Insight into our place and work in this Great Reality, spurs us on. Great Reality is richer than fiction and fantasy. Process is richer than "ready-made" and truer to the adventures of living.

The more I am willing to live life as it is given to me -- with its wonders, dullness, learning, excitement, and satisfaction from working well with others -- the more I "wake-up." I look at the raw materials of life and use them.

May I set realistic self-defined attainable goals. My successes don't come as immediately or quickly as I want. I value them because they come from the raw materials of life. I worked for them.

FOR TODAY: There are satisfactions from achieved competencies, valuing myself and others.

UNLOCKING MY VISIONS   OCTOBER 13

am no longer a slave to dieting and overeating cycles. Yet I am still partly enslaved. I need a Power greater than myself to help me develop my realizable dreams, and work for them. It is good to have a dream. It keeps me moving forward.

FOR TODAY: I am restored to the basic goodness of life.

*"I lost that connection with my original hopes. They were crushed.
I have to go rediscover my authentic self. I have to go deeper. My
Higher Power, or God as I understand him, has got to get bigger.
My Sponsor tells me that is what Step Eleven is for."*
                    --Anonymous

There may have been many ways our original hopes were crushed.
We didn't get the immediate recognition for our talents. There
wasn't the money or glory we hoped for. We didn't have a Plan B. We
lost a job. We didn't get the promotion we had worked for. Our family
situation wasn't what we wanted.

We wished to be moral and kind. Wrong motives and imaginings got
in the way.

My authentic self has been covered up by disappointment turned to
resentment. I may have said my family situation, lack of family or
disruption in romance or marriage was the cause of my troubles.
I may have felt I could not move beyond this disappointment or any
other condition that caused me grief or suffering.

My authentic self has the ability to develop. I have the ability to move
beyond beliefs such as 'Others hold the key to my happiness, destiny
or identity.' Or 'I can't be happy unless a specific event takes place.'
This puts dependence in the wrong place. It ties my happiness to a
limited outcome. I no longer rely on any one human being. I am God
dependent. God has a plan and a purpose for my growth. I realize my
Higher Power is my Source.

In prayer and meditation I tap into spiritual resources. Enthusiastic
again, clear of wrong motives and imaginings, abstinent from diet
substances and compulsive dieting, I get acquainted with my authentic
self. There is a real person here, with real hopes.

FOR TODAY: I pray and meditate to tap into my authentic self.

he only way I can build on identity is to live life. I draw on a Power greater than myself.

A loving God as I understand him wants a full life for each of us. Drawing on this power, we can leave home, metaphorically speaking. We can explore new areas or go beyond our comfort or deprivation zone. We become able to move toward the things that are satisfying to each of us individually and away from those that are not. We become free, also, to succeed.

I am out of vagueness. I focus on good, possible, attainable, spiritual and material goods right for me -- activities - contributions - sensations - merits - thoughts - observations.

We can attend meetings. The Debtors Anonymous fellowship deals with debting, underearning, and building financial and material security. Co-Dependents Anonymous is a fellowship that deals with relationships and how to detach or set boundaries so we may focus on our own essential needs. Al-Anon is a fellowship that deals with living with or interacting with an alcoholic or other substance abuser or person addicted.

Program and fellowship can be an active testing ground to identify goals, spending plans, education or work plans. We can use action partners or sponsors to discuss creative projects. We hear others share their experience, strength and hope in dealing with living issues.

FOR TODAY: I call on new resources.

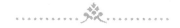

"Vision work is a new idea to me. It gives me permission. It asks me to do the work - to extend my vision - beyond the status quo."
--Anonymous

We have taken steps to obtain new knowledge about ourselves as we are. It is time now to move forward to new behaviors and satisfactions. It is time to do Vision Work. My dreams, daydreams, reveries, and hopes -- My Visions - are part of the raw materials of creation.

"Vision Work" is different from compulsing on "unsatisfied desires." "Vision Work" is not fantastic wishful thinking or daydreaming for ready-mades.

"Vision Work" is active. It puts the "thinking cap" on. It works with reality. What is in front of me? What is in my deepest heart's desire as part of my identity? What visions can I work on? What visions will give me deep satisfactions in working for them? What visions are worth working for? A whole book could be spent on "Doing the Vision Work."

What would I like to happen in my spiritual and material life? What are my materials -- my talents, abilities and God-given enthusiasms? What would I like to do to develop and use my talents, abilities and God-given enthusiasms? What would I like to happen in my relationships with others?

FOR TODAY: Doing this Vision Work is positive and uplifting. I do vision work. What are my visions? What are my goals with the person I am today?

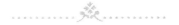

"I got a Pressure Relief Group in Debtors Anonymous to help me develop ideas. I got an Action Partner in Debtors Anonymous to help me take the actions to get a job. It works." --Anonymous

"I recognized I wanted to make $4000. more a year, the amount I would have gotten from a promotion that didn't happen. I had done all this work and wasn't being promoted. I have started a small business. I am making the $4000." --Anonymous

Doing this vision work draws on a Power greater than myself. I am willing to work with others and to ask for their help. They help me think with vision about moving toward my good. Because my vision is values-based, it will be constructive. It will be to my good and to the good of others.

Committing actions to an "action partner" or sponsor is a tool. I commit actions, such as phone calls I need to make, research I need to do to find information on something, shopping for the right stuff. I discuss the emotional hurdles to take the actions. Then I am more ready to take the action. Sometimes I break the action down into steps, and further baby steps, so I don't get frustrated. Then I don't lose sight of my ability to do the action.

FOR TODAY: This vision work includes expanding, squeezing, modifying, shifting, opening, closing, kitchen table finance, psychology, higher level thinking, hope, faith, enjoyment. I have new perceptions. Where there were walls, there are now windows and doors. I open my vision to good things that are possible for me and my world.

onnecting to my enthusiasms connects me to sights, sounds, colors, textures, nature, culture, other people, where I live, and life.

"A start-up enthusiasm -- to get out on the water -- set me on a path of discovery. Starting came after a long delay, illness, and waiting on others. I now know more about the world than when I started... I loved learning about sailing and sailing with the instructor in a Red Cross sailing course. He sailed by angles and visual projections of where he wanted to be. It was not at all like driving a car in lanes... Then, as a volunteer crew on the Clearwater Environmental Sloop, we were on the Hudson River for three days, slept on the sloop, sailing when the outgoing tides would let us go downriver. I hooked up with The Riverkeeper Project where we started to take water samples to build an information database on the river water. My teammate, a science professor, let me sit in on his course in Human Evolution. I read 'The Voyage of The Beagle' about Charles Darwin's boat trip around South America where he got many of his ideas from studying the geography and collecting natural specimens. Then I followed an interest reading Edward O. Wilson's, 'Biodiversity' and 'Naturalist,' Stephen Jay Gould's 'Rocks of Ages: Science and Religion in the Fullness of Life,' and David Sloan Wilson's 'Evolution for Everybody'... I'm uplifted to learn about the organizations of life. There are wonderful things operating - greater things operating than what I know. I'm grateful for the operands of evolution that have created homo sapiens as social and because we are social as a species, an ethic has been created of sharing and cooperation with sanctions against lawbreakers, cheats, thieves, bullies, and murderers; and altruism so that our sharing and treatment of goodness goes beyond kin. The movement of social species is toward stability as it encounters changing conditions." --Anonymous

FOR TODAY: Starting rocks! Just starting. I commit to one of my enthusiasms. The enthusiasm connects me to my energy core and to the world. It is outgoing. I don't worry about an end result.

"My experience has been that when I am following my God-given enthusiasms and seeking to apply them, to follow and develop them, and to serve with them in the world, right work will be on my path. Suzanne Langer in 'Mind: An Essay on Human Feeling' says 'entrainment is the process of individuation. Small acts are gathered into larger acts and carried along.' My dreams and delights from childhood, and constructive play, are now carried forward with real purpose, as I seek outlets to use my delights and talents in the world." --Anonymous

What comes first, the chicken or the egg? Do we commit to our enthusiasms or to core activities first or to everything at the same time?

One thing is certain, recovering our dreams and visions, our authentic enthusiasms, shows recovery from 'diethead' thinking. This movement shows Twelve Step Recovery. For we are now thinking about what our Maker has created, our God-given talents and the world we live in, and how we can use these talents and enthusiasms in the world.

FOR TODAY: I think about what my Maker has created, my God-given talents and the world I live in with others, and how I can use these talents and enthusiasms in the world.

Our need for material security is surely God-given. And our means to adapt to conditions as they are and assume an effective attitude to secure our material well-being is God-given too.

Spiritual progress will diminish my fears that I will be destitute. It will temper the greedy hand. Spiritual progress will give pause to the desire for quick results. It puts priorities in the right order.

FOR TODAY: Today I use the talents God has given me to be in the world the right way.

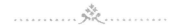

ourage does not always make big noise. It speaks with responsiveness, deliberation and attention to purpose and the welfare of people. Planning actions helps us fill our day with good things and avoid self pity, self-loathing, or any other unmanageable emotions. *"Those who fail to plan, plan to fail"* is a saying often used in Overeaters Anonymous.

Having a food plan, using it daily, planning what will be on it, and knowing the contents and whereabouts of the meals, makes me feel cared for, supported, and guilt free. Planning takes the power out of the food.

The planning keeps me away from diet remedy thinking. There is only need to take essential action - I have meals planned in front of me. Specific, manageable, attainable actions can be envisioned, planned, and carried through. If an action seems too big or difficult, I break it down into smaller actions.

We don't always have the ability to plan. However, we can use our method on planning and taking courageous humble actions with the right motive so that it becomes a thought-process. Thinking 'Humble Actions' gives me perspective on myself, my abilities, what is possible. Thinking 'Courageous Actions' points me in the right direction to live with deliberation.

"...I wanted to live deliberately," Henry David Thoreau wrote. I too am living deliberately. I am opening to the creative Universe. My Higher Power helps me live deliberately. I live with vision.

FOR TODAY: I am living beyond 'diethead' thinking or 'reactiveness.' I am going beyond the passive.

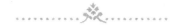

"*My Sister-in-Law raises children and grandchildren.   She laughs with them, disciplines them so they learn about the world and don't get hurt. She feeds them and attends to their needs...*

My Sponsor photographs.   She asks when she bumps into people 'Hi, How 'Ya doing'.   She carries her camera and takes pictures before and after Meetings -- flowering trees - doorways - Christmas decorations...

I quilt. It took me years to start. When I was a young girl I opened a closet and saw a red-white and blue quilt. Wow! 'I want to do that.' I pay someone to cut fabric pieces; this jump starts a project. A group of church ladies quilts the tops. They use their sewing skills; their church gets the quilting fee. I love pouring over fabric catalogs. I like creating the blocks, using lights, mediums and darks. I like sewing blocks by hand, especially sitting outdoors. Members of my family and friends get quilts."
                                        --Anonymous

"*My Mother quilts in her church sewing circle. Her church sends the quilts to the troops...*

I write plays.   I am so grateful I get to hear my words.   I am learning about acceptance. I am learning about the right actor or actress for the right part." --Anonymous

 e can all do something wonderful.

For Today: What is the wonderful thing I do? I smile. There is more than one.

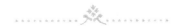

"Character contributes to beauty. It fortifies a woman as her youth fades. A mode of conduct, a standard of courage, discipline, fortitude and integrity can do a great deal to make a woman beautiful." --Jacqueline Bisset, Actress

"Careful grooming may take 20 years off a woman's age, but you can't fool a long flight of stairs." --Marlene Dietrich, Actress

"Beauty is in the eye of the beholder, and it may be necessary from time to time to give a stupid or misinformed beholder a black eye."
--Miss Piggy, Muppet

"Beauty is a characteristic of a person, place, object, or idea that provides a perceptual experience of pleasure, meaning, or satisfaction. Beauty is studied as part of aesthetics, sociology, social psychology, and culture. As a cultural creation, beauty has been extremely commercialized. An "ideal beauty" is an entity which is admired, or possesses features widely attributed to beauty in a particular culture." --Wikipedia

"There is no cosmetic for beauty like happiness."
--Author Unknown

"We are beautiful." --Christina Aguilara, Singer-Singwriter

C ontributing to beauty, we have choices. Physical attractiveness comes from physical health. We have a choice to radiate beauty and self-confidence from physical health, lived values and achieved competencies. We have a choice to radiate beauty, from self-knowledge, our knowledge of what we contribute to life.

FOR TODAY: We are so beautiful.

⁘

"God, Give each of us the awareness that as we work in the world with people, at the desk or computer, as we weigh evaluations in the business world, as we create, in design, or music, or writing, or contribute to the raising of children, we are building these moments into the vast structure of the creative Universe."
                    --Kenneth O. Jones, Minister & Writer

 touch the lives of many. Many touch my life.

FOR TODAY: I have an awareness I exist. I contribute.

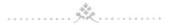

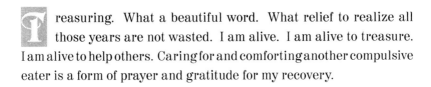 reasuring. What a beautiful word. What relief to realize all those years are not wasted. I am alive. I am alive to treasure. I am alive to help others. Caring for and comforting another compulsive eater is a form of prayer and gratitude for my recovery.

My experience is not wasted. I don't need to expose it in extravagent tale-telling. Because I carry my experience with me, I can use it as a guidepost for living and guiding others. One definition of art is "felt life."

FOR TODAY: I bring "felt life" into my dealings with others. May I bring my feeling for compassion and kindness, endearing humor and hope, tolerance and love.

"Go confidently in the direction of your dreams. Live the life you have imagined." --Henry David Thoreau, Writer

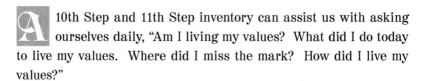 10th Step and 11th Step inventory can assist us with asking ourselves daily, "Am I living my values? What did I do today to live my values. Where did I miss the mark? How did I live my values?"

Usually, every day shows ways I live my values.

Upon awakening, I express gratitude for the new day. I get up to meet the day. I wash and dress for my own appearance and because attention to my appearance shows self-esteem and makes others feel good about my hygiene and grooming. It shows health. I plan and enjoy my food because food is a great good. I talk civilly to the people around me, including my loved ones, neighbors, the bus drivers, the store clerks, people at work.

FOR TODAY:
Giving the perfect smile goes on my list.
Doing service in ways I have chosen.
Using my intelligence and abilities.
Contributing to someone else's well-being and peace.
Being honest.
Valuing others as well as myself.

All of these things are ways of living my values.

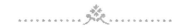

"You don't make friends. You take hostages." –Anonymous

What would I like to happen in my relationships with others? First I have to envision what a true partnership with another human being might be. I realize what I have in mind may not be a true partnership at all. My imagination calls up fantasies where the other person does not exist at all. They are invisible – they do everything I want magically. Perhaps I envision a Higher Power that makes the other person do everything I want. That is a misperception of Higher Power. Perhaps I envision a partnership where I am invisible - and I expect the other person to be a mind reader and magically read and grant my wishes. That is not a partnership at all.

Either I want to control and dominate, or I want the other person to. I want to ride on the coattails of the other person. They "owe" me for my loyalty I think. I want them to satisfy me. Or I am in denial about who they really are. Fantasizing is not "envisioning."

It takes maturity to form a true partnership with another human being. We may have many true partnerships – with neighbors, family, loved ones, a special someone, co-workers, employees, bosses, doctors, care providers.

In a partnership, both parties exist. Both parties are in the field, in the play, in the arena, bring something to the table. Neither dominates, though each may have their strengths and specialties. Each are themselves; they are not a mirror copy of the other.

We want balance. We want to be "right size". We want to carry our weight, each as we are able. We do not rescue or caretake. We are aware of our own expectations of being rescued or caretaked and let go of them. Love is based on maturity and responsibility for self and giving freely what we are able.

FOR TODAY: May I remember others in my life are uniquely themselves. They are not my possessions. Others have their own Higher Power. Envisioning what is right in relatedness helps me bring it into practice and being.

TOLERATING HUMAN FRAILTIES - MINE TOO   OCTOBER 28

y identity becomes larger when I can tolerate human frailties.

People are all different. People do not think alike. People have not seen the same things, listened to the same music, seen the same TV shows, read the same books. People are in different generations. People have different experiences.

What I perceive as "human frailty" may in fact be only these differences between people. How someone acts may go against my assumptions, based on what I would do or how I think.

When I build on identity, I open myself to the world and the true differences between people. "What do you think?" I ask. Appreciating someone's thought or behavior, I don't have to dominate. I can make a realistic appraisal of myself and others. We all have good days and bad days.

FOR TODAY: I understand we all have good days and bad days.

"Today I identify the biggest red leaf on the nearest pin oak tree. My tea with lemon is especially delicious." --Anonymous

"Looking at my Peanuts collection of Charles Schulz cartoons brings a smile to my face. I look at it at bedtime. It brings me into my humanity. Kids sure have frustration. I am inspired to think humorously about the human condition. And to put some of this into my work." --Anonymous

I am a person who has sprung free and has emotional mobility. I am able to move toward the things that are satisfying to me and away from those that are not. I am free also, to succeed. I move toward satisfying meals. Food is a great good to be used in its goodness. I focus on good, possible, attainable activities - contributions - merits - observations. It might be something simple. It might be something complicated, with many parts. Life is not without its complications, foils, thwarted efforts. We all deal with frustrations.

Today I respect the time it takes to be in a long-term relationship, to build social skills, to build skills on a job or to build a career or profession. It takes a big investment purpose to raise a child. For all these things it takes tenacity, perseverance, and a right heart.

FOR TODAY: I am able to move toward the things that are satisfying to me and away from those that are not.

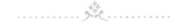

"Lord, make me a channel of thy peace, that where there is hatred, I may bring love--that where there is wrong, I may bring the spirit of forgiveness--that where there is discord, I may bring harmony--that where there is error, I may bring truth--that where there is doubt, I may bring faith--that where there is despair, I may bring hope--that where there are shadows, I may bring light--that where there is sadness, I may bring joy. Lord, grant that I may seek rather to comfort than to be comforted--to understand, than to be understood--to love, than to be loved. For it is by self-forgetting that one finds. It is by forgiving that one is forgiven. It is by dying that one awakens to Eternal Life. Amen."

--The St. Francis Prayer

In a time of shifting values, I can have despair thoughts. I can be aware of the bad, the wrong, the sordid or the mean, the horrid, the sorrowful, the tragic. I can be aware when things just don't make sense.

Preserving noble standards in a time of shifting values is one way I consciously build on my identity. When despair and cynicism crop up, I am aware of it. With the help of my Higher Power, I practice positive actions. I hope to provide assurance to others that I am fair, and that in other arenas right will prevail over wrong. Higher Power works through many people.

May I move beyond despair and help others move beyond despair to a full life. In this way I preserve noble standards. I replace any despair thoughts and doubt with kind actions and thoughts.

FOR TODAY: I am kind. I pray for healing of body, mind and spirit. I pray this for myself. I pray it for others.

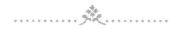

"I am a playright. By having my work read at open workshops, I network with actors and actresses and other playrights."
--Anonymous

"Work has an element of play because I'm on teams and work projects with others. Sometimes there are shifting teams with different members. I enjoy it. How do I want to play? I want to play with others, not alone." --Anonymous

ach day is precious to me. Each 24 hours. How do I want to play? It is not only a matter of what is presented before me from the media. To the contrary, I must ask my true self "how do I want to play?" What would I enjoy? What would give me pleasure?

"Play is the work of children."
--Friedrich Froebel, Toy Designer & Childhood Educator

One of the highest activities of humanity is play. Different games provide different types of interaction. Tennis is a highly competitive game between two people. Solitary play helps idea formation in children. Play with others - one person, two people, team play, even shifting teams as in a work setting, requires and builds social skills.

I have to wear different hats, play as a team and play on many teams. There are some modes I don't have to play in if I don't enjoy it. I don't have to play with "entertainment" that is put passively in front of me if that is not true play for me. I can enjoy doing something satisfying to me personally.

For Today: I choose satisfying play.

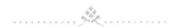

y ego, intelligence, heredity, matter and spirit, education, and repetitive measures, do not give me complete control over my body chemistry or formation processes. Nor would I want them to. What a job! LIFE is greater than this.

I let go of highs or lows or compulsions from compulsive overeating or dieting. At first these things gave me an excitement, a thrill or a buzz or a sense I was accomplishing something. Then they turned on me. I was accomplishing nothing of worth. It was smoke, not warmth from the fire.

FOR TODAY: May I take joy and satisfaction in my Creation. My life is manageable because I respect life. I have spiritual principles guiding me.

he most common compulsive overeater's fantasy is "If I just lose weight, everything will be alright."

Even with food plans and the best planning, I will experience discomfort, upsets, and uncertainty, as well as ordinary days with unpredictable encounters.

May I practice emotional stability to temper rage, frustration or disappointment. May I practice loving-kindness.

FOR TODAY: The fog has lifted. I leave the fantasy and live in reality.

When I am having a difficult time accepting myself as I am, I work on humility. I regain my humanity. I am human, not perfect. I ask for the willingness to be honest, and let this be the true me I let others see. I accept my physical self, for now.

FOR TODAY: I work a program to be the best me I can be. I exist. I am a flesh and blood person.

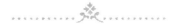

"So while I think of it,
let me paint a thank-you on my palm
for this God, this laughter of the morning,
lest it go unspoken.
The Joy that isn't shared, I've heard,
dies young."
--Anne Sexton, Poet

A thankful heart won't be a resenting heart. Each morning I start out thanking God for my mind and myself for using the mind God gave me.

FOR TODAY: I have a full and thankful heart.

"The lunatic, the lover, and the poet
Are of imagination all compact:
One sees more devils than vast hell can hold,
That is, the madman: the lover, all as frantic,
Sees Helen's beauty in a brow of Egypt:
The poet's eye, in a fine frenzy rolling,
Doth glance from heaven to earth, from earth to heaven;
And as imagination bodies forth
The forms of things unknown, the poet's pen
Turns them to shapes, and gives to airy nothing
A local habitation and a name.
Such tricks hath strong imagination,
That if it would but apprehend some joy,
It comprehends some bringer of that joy;
Or in the night, imagining some fear,
How easy is a bush supposed a bear!"
--William Shakespeare, *A Midsummer's Night Dream*

L etting go of folly, fear, lunacy, and grandiose expectations opens the door to new vistas, set on right objectives, using "constructive imagination".

I can accomplish good things. My objectives are important. Am I kind? Do I have an ethic of respect?

For Today: I use constructive imagination.

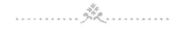

"This recent visit to my doctor was so helpful. We talked, again, as many times, about the latest diet program I heard about. She explained to me how dangerous the weight loss method was. Then we talked about my eating and exercise patterns. She endorsed me for my good choices that are leading to low blood pressure and good HDL cholesterol. We talked about weight loss that will keep to my decision to abstain from diet drugs and compulsive dieting. I will continue to make good food choices, work with my OA Sponsor, and monitor portions. I came away feeling good. My life is manageable. Weight management is possible."

--Anonymous

I t is alright to talk to my doctor about weight loss. I am not anti-doctor or against medicines. However, there is a fact -- I have abused diet drugs and food. My life-enhancing decision to let go of compulsive overeating and weight loss methods involving drugs needs to be foremost in my communication with my doctor. My doctor can work with me for my physical and mental health by having complete information about me. I let my doctor know my background, my experience, my susceptibilities to drug abuse, and my decisions.

Like the recovering alcoholic, some of us compulsive eaters have misused drugs, often as a substitute for other physical, emotional and spiritual solutions to our problems of living. We have misused drugs in such a manner as to become a threat to the achievement and maintenance of abstinence and clean and sober living.

I find the ideas expressed in the *A.A.Conference Approved Statement on Drug Use* helpful. To paraphrase – I am aware of the misuse of drugs. At the same time, just as it would be wrong to enable or support anyone to become re-addicted to a drug, it would be wrong to deprive anyone of a necessary medication which can alleviate or control other disabling physical and or mental problems. Some people must take prescribed medication in order to treat certain serious medical problems. I find these suggestions helpful to guide me:

1. I will remember that as a person recovering from misuse of weight loss methods involving drugs and compulsive overeating my automatic response will be to turn to chemical relief for uncomfortable feelings. I will look for non-chemical solutions for the aches and discomforts of everyday living.

2. I will remember that the best safeguard against a diet substance drug-related relapse is an active participation in the Twelve Step Programs of Recovery.

3. I remember that no Twelve Step Program member plays Doctor. The meditations in this reader are not intended to diagnose or treat or cure any illness and do not constitute medical advice. Consult your physician for medical advice.

4. I am completely honest with myself and my physician regarding use of medication.

5. I consult a physician with demonstrated experience in the treatment of drug addiction, and with the abuses of diet substances and compulsive dieting, and with awareness of the problems associated with use of diet substances, diet remedies, and compulsive dieting.

6. I am honest about my use of diet substances and compulsive dieting with any physician I consult. Such knowledge is important to my doctor.

7. I ask my doctor to give careful consideration to any treatment methods for any conditions, given my experience and problems with use of diet substances and compulsive dieting.

8 . I inform the physician at once if I experience side effects from prescribed drugs.

9. For me, the decision to take medication should be made primarily between a doctor who is informed about my experience and problems with use of diet substances and compulsive dieting and a patient, me, who is informed about the medication.

WORKING A PROGRAM

10. I believe it is important for anyone who is considering taking medication to get as much information as possible before taking it.

11. I consider consulting another doctor if a personal physician refuses or fails to recognize the peculiar susceptibility of me to sedatives, tranquilizers, and stimulants, diet substances or compulsive dieting methods.

12. I believe that, just as it is wrong to enable or support anyone to become re-addicted to any drug or type of drug they have had problems with and do not decide to take, it is equally wrong to deprive anyone of a necessary medication which can alleviate or manage other physical and or mental problems.

FOR TODAY: I have a deeper understanding of the pill problem. The experience of others and my own experience puts this guiding light before me as I live my life.

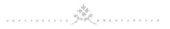

LETTING HIGHER POWER LEAD   NOVEMBER 7

"Lead by getting out of the way." --Lao Tzu, Philosopher

I am surrendered to doing my part. I get out of the way of my own recovery. There is a Higher Power at work here, a sunshine of the Spirit. When things come up I respond as needed.

FOR TODAY: May I bask in the light and breathe the good air today.

"The last time I went to a new doctor, because my regular doctor was out of town, she offered 'We can give you something to lose weight.' I refused it. I knew it was bad medicine. She had not taken a medical history. She made faulty assumptions about blood pressure, blood cholesterol and blood sugar. I had gone to be treated for a respiratory infection." –Anonymous

Staying clear of diet drugs or other methods of dieting compulsively is as easy or as hard as I make it. I can get off the merry-go-round. Or I can go round and round. I can make someone an expert or dominant over my life. I can be dependent and assume someone knows all about managing my life. Or I can assume responsibility for my life with my Higher Power. Being honest about what is and isn't a diet substance for me helps.

I keep going back to this -- is this a diet substance? Is this going to start a pattern of compulsion again? Are the expectations here magical expectations? Am I turning away, deciding against trust in my Higher Power and wise-mind?

God, help me stay honest. In times of confusion, doubt or frustration. let me remember this is a good time to have trust and faith. Let me remember there is clear thought and vision. I have tapped into this wise-mind before and I will tap into it again. It is never lost.

FOR TODAY: I have a Higher Power.

"No matter what happens, keep on beginning and failing. Each time you fail, start all over again, and you will grow stronger until you find that you have accomplished a pupose-not the one you began with perhaps, but one you will be glad to remember."
--Anne Sullivan, Teacher

 here are lots of reasons that might drive me to relapse:

1. Someone started a diet program and lost weight. Maybe they are the example? I question myself. I've lost my boundaries. I forget that I'm an individual with my own path, not co-dependent. I take responsibility for my own life. I'm an example in the world with my physical, emotional and spiritual recovery. I am well, and not obsessed, and am able to help and serve others.

2. Self-loathing has kicked in. I want an easy and quick make-over. I want to re-invent myself and think a relapse with diet substances and compulsive dieting might do it. I'll get a new romance. I'll never get old.

3. I forget that not using "alcohol'" [food or diet products and methods] is only a beginning on dealing with life problems.

4. A new diet product came out on the market. I see the ads on TV and in the magazines. They have movie stars and pop singers raving about their weight loss benefits on the substance.

5. A new trigger food came out on the market. I don't want to be left out. I forget that it is the same old stuff packaged a new way, with a new promise, that is a lie. It will not deliver happiness or safety.

6. I want immediate gratification. I'll do anything to escape the aversion to where I am now emotionally. I have to react. It is where I have a "mental blank spot" or instant forgetter about what compulsive overeating does to me.

It is where I blank out my history. It is where I think trigger foods, or purging, starving, taking metabolizers, fat blockers, carb blockers, central nervous stimulants, appetite suppressants, diet drugs, laxatives, diuretics, exercising compulsively, or any of the methods I have tried will make me feel better, distract me from present pain, and solve my problems. It is where I think - I'm at the end of my rope. In Twelve Step Recovery they say, "When you get to the end of your rope, tie a knot and hang on."

FOR TODAY: Thinking critically about what compulsive eating does to me helps avoid relapse.

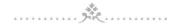

BEING KNOCKED OFF CENTER
GETTING CENTERED AGAIN   NOVEMBER 10

"You have found your path and it is healthy and right for you. You have been able to come out of it much faster and easier these days - that is great growth." --Anonymous

Another person's burdens with food, nutrition, diet and weight can knock me off center. Being knocked off center and getting centered again is a recovery process. I call on my Higher Power, and the help of other people. My life is not my own but belongs to all the people who have helped me.

Living my life effectively involves using all my skills -- recovery from diet substance use and compulsive dieting, recovery from overeating and undereating, recovery from co-dependence, to respect and re-set my boundaries, with the ability to take care of myself, living in integrity.

FOR TODAY: I am centered on my path.

At first I took diet substances and dieted compulsively because I wanted a smaller waist size and number on the scale. That was my purpose - and to get everything I thought the waist size and scale number would bring. Demoralized I stumbled through the doors of Overeaters Anonymous. I had experienced repeated frustration and torture on my purpose.

I have been given hope and dignity. I have been given much more - clarity and direction for my life. It feels liberating to let go of my limited perspective. My body parts are not the center of the world. Health is a purpose. Playing my part in contributing and being of service is a purpose.

FOR TODAY: The scale or the measuring tape is not the yardstick of my purpose.

"I have heard people say 'I want the physical recovery.' Some Sponsors sponsor only for weight loss. Wanting the physical recovery alone is probably a limited objective. With right living and right thinking my physical recovery comes. I am on a new footing. There is a new purpose to my recovery and to me."
                    --Anonymous

Today I work a program for physical recovery with a right heart and my wise-mind. I am not the same person I was. All my recovery is with me. I am diligent about taking proper nutrition and exercise. I have presence of mind - peace of mind. I am not compulsive. I am not going to beat the world.

FOR TODAY: I am not desperate. I am a person of grace and dignity.

"Today I humbly ask my Higher Power for the grace to find the space between my impulse and my action; to let flow the cooling breeze when I would respond with heat; to interrupt fierceness with gentle peace; to accept the moment which allows judgment to become discernment; to defer to silence when my tongue would rush to attack or defend." --Reflections, Alcoholics Anonymous

"...we pause, when agitated or doubtful, and ask for the right thought or action." --Alcoholics Anonymous, Third Edition

I temper instincts and let my drives be restored to their true purpose. In Steps Ten and Eleven, I raise my heart and mind to God, praying for right things of which I am in need and others are in need.

FOR TODAY: May I put a thought between my impulse and my action. Is this the right action I want to take? Living on the basis of a clean house and body, not delusions, fabrications, or distorted drives, God permits me to be a gracious person.

MAKING DECISIONS VS. REACTING   NOVEMBER 14

Today I make decisions and act on them, rather than reacting to people, what they are doing, what they say. I was way too overreactive. I don't take the "bait". I am not a reactive fish. I am a human being with a big brain that God gave me to use. *"...For after all God gave us our brains to use." --Alcoholics Anonymous*, Third Edition.

May I set my course with the food and meals through the day. I practice emotional sobriety. I don't have to jump on anyone's diet bandwagon. The emotional power of the food slips away because I have emotional sobriety.

FOR TODAY: I have presence of mind.

y keeping my memory green I turn my troubling experience into helpful awareness, to bring it in a quiet way to the newcomer or next struggling compulsive overeater. Abstinent now for several years, I am grateful for God's love and the help I have received in the fellowship.

FOR TODAY: I don't live in the past. I am forward helping.

HAVING GOOD FUN   NOVEMBER 16

"Law Office humor - 'I'm up to my neck in alligators.' 'Did yours get fed yet?' Joking around perks up my spirits and the other person's too." --Anonymous

"Life itself is the proper binge." --Julia Child, Chef & Writer

efore my recovery, everything was so serious. Self-pity and power-driven willfulness denied me ordinary fun. Today, I live life to the fullest. I laugh when people make jokes. I find I'm pretty funny myself. I laugh with others.

I can tell about my spiritual and emotional state by where my humor goes. If it is bitter, it means I'm bitter, or tired, or depleted. If it is mean or sordid, I may be slipping. Awareness coaxes me to listen to my Higher Power and do a spot-check inventory. By looking at what I'm bitter or angry about, I can turn to my Higher Power and ask what can I do about it? How can prayer and meditation lighten my load, relieve my burden, or change my outlook? How can rest and self-care restore my resources? How can sharing with another person provide comfort and assurance and change my bitter perspective?

FOR TODAY: Joking around will be fun today. Everything has its right place and purpose.

"For it is by self-forgetting that one finds."
                                        --The St. Francis Prayer

I t is a good feeling to care about somebody else, to know what they are feeling. I have always had the capacity for caring. However, I never knew how to care before without being swamped by other people's burdens. Or I felt I was terminally unique with my burdens.

Everybody has something -- some troubles, some abilities, some beauties. Their trouble is not my trouble. I learn about others. I see where I begin and end. I listen actively. When I pay attention to someone else, they know it and feel heard. Listening actively creates trust in the room. Everyone is listening. It's the same respect I get.

Shifting the focus away from myself helps me feel useful. By listening to others who have purged, binged, and experienced compulsive overeating and or undereating, I recognize similarities. We admit that the chips are down. We are sick and suffering.

FOR TODAY: Paying attention to someone else helps me. I am part of the Universe. The Universe has ears.

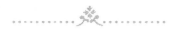

I am in a state of wakefulness. One day at a time, trigger foods or foods in excessive amounts or diet products or methods are not for me. It's not for me, whatever it is. I am relieved of opinion.

While I am in a state of wakefulness, my ears and mind can jump. What is this? What is this new thing? What does it have to offer? My heart beats faster. I am like an animal who has sighted something move. The brain's sense of adventure has kicked in. Let me not jump off a cliff chasing a dry bone.

FOR TODAY: I am relieved of opinion and impulse when it comes to jumping for trigger foods. May I keep my memory green on this.

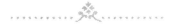

Self-loathing vanishes. I have tapped an inner resource.

I have a choice between self-respect and self-loathing. I can choose integrity and not despair. I can choose love and not hate. I can choose self-centered isolation. Or perhaps I will choose solitude and cloistering. Isolation and solitude are two different things. I can renew my resources and enter the world in confidence.

FOR TODAY: May I see myself in a good light.

I don't know what will happen exactly as I practice letting go of compulsive eating and diet products and methods. Today, I am abstinent from these behaviors -- not eating, liquid fasts, appetite suppressants, central nervous system stimulants, diet boosters, diet blasters, diet blockers, metabolizers, diet bitter herbs, diet herbal teas, diet powders, diet liquids, diet pills, diuretics, purging, laxatives, punishing exercise, prescription drugs, over the counter drugs, compulsive exercise or combinations and variations of all of them. I believe I can live in health without them.

Trusting and holding on, I hold on to my decision and trust God to walk with me this road to recovery. It takes me on a satisfying road, to be lived well each day.

The mud puddles of yesterday are in different places today. There are new challenges. New answers will come. I move beyond "diethead". I choose the life-enhancing.

God, What lies in the great unknown beyond compulsive eating? You created me to grow and mature. My body will go through different changes and change shapes at different times during my life. Let me rely on the growth and maturing process you have established in my biology, during all the stages of my life, to live in health and wisdom. Let me respect the goodness and rightness of food. Let me eat food in the right amounts. There are Twelve Step Programs and Sponsors to help me deal with eating issues. Let me rely on Your Power for my health and well-being.

FOR TODAY: New answers come. Today will show me ways I am well-made. It will be a delight.

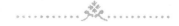

nger is an insanity I cannot afford. It comes in many faces – scorny face, frowny face, bitterness, jealousy. Sometimes I cannot even see the face – my own angry face. Anger can ruin a day, a week, a month, a year, or more. Before the Twelve Step Program unidentified bitterness overlaid every moment.

I can be blinded by anger. Sometimes expressing it to another person, I see the anger, the emotion, apart from the subject it is about. Then I realize how anger is an emotional color – red! I can be emotionally sober when I listen to another person tell me about their anger. Since their anger does not involve me, I see them and the anger and can understand or counsel if asked.

Since recovery, I see the good in the world and in me. With gratitude, I have little to be angry about. I have been blessed.

FOR TODAY: I am blessed. I let go of anger to lift the fog from my eyes. I wipe my eyes to see the blessings.

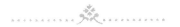

he impulse to do something can be blocked by fear. Maybe we haven't done what we want before. Maybe we are afraid to start. Talking about it with our Sponsor or another trusted person can help. It puts the fear right out in front on the table. Then we can see what actions we might need to take.

FOR TODAY: I am willing to express my fear to a trusted person. I am willing to walk toward good things

The Serenity Prayer asks us to acknowledge what we can and cannot do. This means acknowledging the abilities of others to do some things I cannot do. When I do this, I don't endanger others by taking on responsibilities I am not qualified to do or wouldn't be good at.

Acknowledging the rights and prerogatives of others shows respect. It shows the right humility to respect others' abilities and talents. I give praise for the abilities of others. Life is large. It takes many people to make a culture.

FOR TODAY: I respect my part. I respect others.

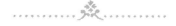

The joy and relief I experience in finding right activities for me is beyond description. I feel free from the bondage of contest. Yet the world is varied enough I can achieve in arenas that are right for me. There is no contest when I am part of the team, the show, the endeavor. I am successful for my part. My contributions are good to the enterprise.

FOR TODAY: I know deep inside I am happy when I seek humility. This means doing well what I do well and knowing what others do well.

I give thanks. Foremost, I don't have to worry about going through a withdrawal from diet products or methods. I will not have future symptoms with troubled thinking or functioning. My head is clear. My body is clean. The satisfaction of not overeating, one meal, one moment, one day at a time, is great. I have the freedom to achieve, to accomplish, and to practice courage. I accept reality and do the best I can do on life's terms and affirm the life enhancing.

FOR TODAY: I am blessed.

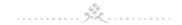

BEING RELIEVED OF THE BONDAGE OF SELF   NOVEMBER 26

When I was overeating compulsively all my thinking was "I" "I" "I" sung to the tune of "Me" "Me" Me". Hideous abjection or hideous conceit. That characterized my soul sickness.

I need to let go of fear, fear of others, fear of lack of love, fear of economic insecurity, and other fears. I need to let go of body criticism. Isolation and self-loathing kept me imprisoned.

The journey to move outward from myself and find my Higher Power began in a recognition of "We." *"We admitted we were powerless over ..."*

The inner critic, the inner tyrant, is often calmed and put to rest as we share. The inner dictatorship is called quits. New self-understanding brings a different response to life's situations.

FOR TODAY: Being relieved of the bondage of self opens me to the world's gifts. Sharing calmly shows me me.

ccepting myself is easier if I acknowledge my life so far by telling somebody else about it.

FOR TODAY: It's ok to be me.

LETTING GO OF GRANDIOSITY
EXPECTATIONS & PRIDE   NOVEMBER 28

I give so much..." was a set up for resentment. Thinking "I give so much..." may express pride. When examined in the light of day, this perception is tempered. Others give too, from their talent base. No wonder they don't see me as "the Great I Am" who gives so much. I may give a lot from my resources. Others may lack appreciation or not show it. I am unable to judge. Judgments, fault-finding and criticism could mean relapse for me. I immediately practice the St. Francis Prayer, *"Lord, make me an instrument of Thy peace; where there is hatred, let me sow love; where there is injury, pardon; where there is doubt, faith; where there is despair, hope; where there is darkness, light; and where there is sadness, joy. O Divine Master, grant that I may not so much seek to be consoled as to console; to be understood, as to understand; to be loved, as to love; for it is in giving that we receive, it is in pardoning that we are pardoned, and it is in dying that we are born to Eternal Life."*

When I let go of grandiosity or pride and reduce expectations, I am less hypersensitive and have less tendency toward resentment. I am less prone to feeling cheated or deprived. In my desires, I often want to make everyone my family – my workplace, my co-workers. I want their approval and love. When I reduce expectations, and get out of denial, I see the situation as it is. My relatedness level is OK.

FOR TODAY: What am I bringing to others freely without an expectation?

"There is a courtesy of the heart; it is allied to love. From it springs the purest courtesy in the outward behavior."
                    --Johann Wolfgang von Goethe, Writer

"Each day I notice how others are gracious to me - how they are kind, how they take time with me, how they talk nicely to me, how they honor me with respect. It is impressive once my perception to notice it opens. I choose to be gracious to others. Going out of my way to say 'no rush,' and to not put people in a rush, to be understanding and forgiving in case of an honest mistake, saying 'that is not a problem. I understand. It could happen to anyone...' Thanking people for their work, saying 'You have been especially helpful. I appreciate it...' Acknowledging others' troubles by saying 'I'm sorry you had that headache...' builds bonds that ease the trouble. Words like this sweeten life. 'Freely have ye received, freely give...'" --Anonymous & The Bible: Matthew 10:8

I am lifted up when I practice courtesy and kindness. I am transported out of myself - yet it is me. The benefits surely set me on the path with a heart. I contribute to the working great stability between people. Culture and harmony make the day joyous. I am joyful.

FOR TODAY: I honor others with kindness and courtesy.

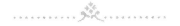

L iving in emotional sobriety and spiritual balance one day at a time allows me to keep focus. I don't want or need to diet compulsively, one day at a time.

I don't kid myself. I could get frenetic, frenzied, worried, upset at any time. I could want to eat compulsively at any time.

FOR TODAY: Emotional sobriety and spiritual balance is a measure of achievement, one day at a time.

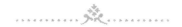

"I watched the seagull. It rose on the power of its anatomy and the air currents. It did what it was made for. There was reliance. There was trust. If it had struggled to hem and haw and miss the day it would have missed life." --Anonymous

 hinking too much, manipulating too much, fearing too much can prevent me from trusting the Power to live.

FOR TODAY: I live this day. The Power of my anatomy, Life, and my Higher Power carries me.

"Beseech you, sir, be merry
So have we all, of joy."
--William Shakespeare, *The Tempest*

 e have come ashore safely. We are in it together - in the sailing, in the tempest, in coming safely ashore. We experience the joy of living.

Being in the solution is a joy. Self-searching is the means by which I bring new vision, action and grace to bear in my life. Learning to use constructive imagination, to build on my identity, and to move toward satisfying activities, I live a full life being in the world. I love the whole pattern of living. I come to terms with failure and success, sickness, or poverty, loneliness or bereavement. I take my problems as they come and do not try to escape. Lesser achievements are granted me along with successes. I have dignity and grace. I am not living in fear. I am made well.

FOR TODAY: I am willing to stay right size. I can give reassurance and support to another compulsive eater that recovery is possible. I can have physical and mental health and help another.

"Having had a spiritual awakening as the result of these steps, we tried to carry this message to others, and to practice these principles in all our affairs." --Step Twelve, The Twelve Steps

"The joy of living is in action and in turning from self-absorption. When did I feel I could get out of myself and enter the world with a Higher Power? When self-centeredness failed me miserably. With small actions, I changed. People appreciated the love and attention I had to give far more than the number I was on the scale or the size pants I wore. My health in the world comes from being functional to contribute. My physical recovery is important to functioning. My spiritual and emotional health is important to it all." --Anonymous

Moving outward, I have a new attention. My mental and physical health, and a spiritual health is greater than diethead. Life has real satisfactions.

FOR TODAY: Moving outward, day by day, I live life. I live in joy.

"It takes at least 50 other human beings to raise a child."
--Sherman Paul, Writer

"It takes a village to raise a child." "Ora na azu nwa""
--Nigerian Proverb
--Adapted for Book Title 'It Takes a Village' by
Hillary Rodham Clinton, U.S. Secretary of State

I seek and accept support from many sources, from the Twelve Step Programs, life teachers, healthcare providers, wise men and women, bosses and co-workers, trusted friends and family. I learn what the accepted practices are. The rules and guidelines have been created for me. When I get to work on time, for example, I am relieved of guilt. I perform better. A baby does not survive without the support of other humans.

FOR TODAY: I see and hear the wisdom others provide. I am not an island unto myself. This is a spiritual awakening worth carrying.

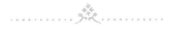

God wants life for me. By removing my gnawing compulsion to compulsively overeat, God has changed my perspective. Reconstructing my life is an important goal in my life.

FOR TODAY: The life force leads me forward into action.

ime used to be my enemy. I was in a hurry. Today I know, the flower doesn't bloom in fast motion. Time is a wonder to behold. It is something great, to be filled with spiritual recovery and appreciated with enthusiasm.

How do I wait when I want so quickly? I have never been known for my patience. When I first came into Twelve Step Recovery I was elated. I thought I had gotten it all in the first few years. Now I practice active patience. I see my life unfold with the principles of spiritual recovery in hand. I appreciate this lifelong task.

I give time time. I give time for growth.

FOR TODAY: Time is my friend. Wherever I am, there I am. I give myself time for growth. I will enjoy this gift today.

he joy of living is in knowing where I begin and where I end. I know what I am Powerless over, and where I have Power. This gives me wisdom.

I have power. I have the power to choose Self-respect over Self-loathing. Integrity over Despair. Love over Hate. Entering the World over Self-centered Isolation. Confidence over Self-pity. I have the power to see the world as an abundant place. My power is not as limited as I once thought. I do not have to go to places or people that do not support or love me. I do not have to go to the diet pill bottles. They are not the choice I want to make today. I have the power to make good choices about food, to plan my meals. I make sure the right food in the right amounts is available to me. I have the power to help others with kindness.

FOR TODAY: I start with deliberate actions. I am strong. I am well made. My efforts are good.

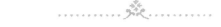

"With joy unfeigned brothers and sisters meet,
And each for other's weelfare kindly spies:
The social hours, swift-winged, unnoticed fleet "
                    --Robert Burns, Poet

t is a miracle to have a path to follow that restores me to sanity. Overeaters Anonymous and other Twelve Step Recovery meetings are a practice space, where I can see what it feels like to be myself. I face my issues with food on new terms. Others are not mobilized against me. At times I have been mobilized against myself. It is a place for me to give up fear.

FOR TODAY: I am accepted by others. This awareness releases energy.

"A graphics person explodes in an email and threatens to quit. I get it. The week before I was upset about everything. I share that. 'It's the middle of winter' I tell her. 'Take it easy.' 'We've had a week of 28 degree weather.' We mend the upset. She says she overreacted. Even on the worst days, I can be in contact with others, in non-hurtful ways. I can share in recognition."

--Anonymous

"When I talk to another compulsive overeater, I'm just enough encouraged that things are not as impossible, or as overwhelming as I thought. My problems are not so unique. They are manageable. My disease is arrested. I plan and get my food. I get up and walk on the hour around the office to get in walking. My disease is arrested."

--Anonymous

I can get the love and understanding I really want and need. It might feel good to be passively dependent, to ride on someone's coattails, or to lean. I still feel insecure at times. Yet I am aware. The people I am leaning on are not holding me up. They are standing next to me.

Companionship lets me know things are not as extreme as they sometimes seem. My isolated thoughts can be chilling. My spirits are warmed by others.

I use the phone, email, and face-to-face conversation. Face-to-face is the best. Popping off erratically in an email is bad for everybody and can cause a lot of problems. I can't hear tone of voice in an email. Hearing someone's voice in person or on the phone is better.

FOR TODAY: I enjoy companionship.

"It would indeed give me a certain household joy to quit this lofty seeking, this spiritual astronomy, or search of stars, and come down to warm sympathies with you..."
        –Ralph Waldo Emerson, Essayist, *"Friendship"*

Growing with others in fellowship is rewarding. We see young men and women come in and leave desperation behind. We see others grow older at my home meeting, face health challenges and yes even pass away being secure in their abstinence. This is holy living as I see it. The most basic kind of daily living with secure peace.

FOR TODAY: I let myself grow with others.

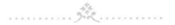

On entering Twelve Step Recovery rooms, I listened to others talk about desperation, unhappiness, and illness as they described their compulsive overeating.

As I listened more, I heard another experience described, the reality of abstinence. It was both an abstinence from diet substances and compulsive dieting methods, and an abstinence from compulsive overeating and undereating.

Daily abstinence means a great deal to me.

FOR TODAY: I listen for the Joy of this Abstinence in meetings. I hear it.

"Made a decision to turn our will and our lives over to the care of God as we understood him."
                    --Step Three, The Twelve Steps

omeone or something chose to preserve me. I choose to believe I have been in God's care. God grants me a number of days in this life until physical death.

God, I cooperate with the forces of health. Your love is a great light, with values of love, conveyed through individuals.

FOR TODAY: If I can be a channel of this love to others - and provide comfort - then I will feel a channel of God's peace.

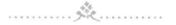

"We are indeed much more than we eat, but what we eat can nevertheless help us to be much more than what we are."
                    --Adele Davis, Nutritionist & Writer

"Salmon from Alaska climb stairs! It's truly amazing how food gets to my table." --Anonymous

ood resumes its proper place in my life. Proper nutrition, regular meals, right food in the right amounts, food as a personal need, and eating as social communion, takes a joyful place in my life today.

FOR TODAY: I enjoy nourishing food. I appreciate all the hands that grow it and bring it to my table. I will relish planning my food, getting it, cooking it, and eating today.

"...and when this is all over, I'll never be hungry again.... Tara!
Home. I'll go home. And I'll think of some way to get him back.
After all.. tomorrow is another day."
     --Vivien Leigh *(as Scarlett O'Hara in Gone With the Wind)*

"Light tomorrow with today." - Elizabeth Barrett Browning, Poet

he best day and the only day I have is TODAY. Living today well is an investment in tomorrow. I know the difference between overzealous compulsive thinking and balanced right thinking. To be secure, I plan my meals. I make sure the food is available to me. This provides me assurance. I am safe.

FOR TODAY: I live in hope. I have comfort. I like my behaviors moment by moment.

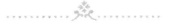

"Finding the love in my eyes and in the eyes of others in fellowship
is part of the joy. This is what I see. My eyes shine with love,
and not with fear. It is a visible sign of Joy. Others too have
love in their eyes and not fear. They know we can leave behind
the desperation involved in taking diet substances and dieting
compulsively. We give one another time to grow." -- Anonymous

We grow in the sunshine of the spirit. Having something to contribute is wealth. True joy. Giving.

FOR TODAY: I put love in my eyes today. At the end of the day, I count five times I saw love in my eyes today.

Self-esteem has to have advancement markers. We advance because we take actions. We *"Humbly ask God to remove our shortcomings."* We don't set a timetable on having character defects removed. *"We continued to take personal inventory..."* We watch for dishonesty, selfishness, pride, grandiosity, and wrong motives. *"Having had a spiritual awakening, we seek to practice these principles in all our affairs..."*

We do advance. Things get better. They get better for us personally. And we build self-esteem as we go along. Where we may have felt "less than" and wanted to be "more than," we claim our humanity. We grow up, to no longer want to dominate or be overly dependent. We want to be self-supporting, rather than live on a handout or ride on someone's coattails. We develop and live our talents. We are relieved of the insane urges to diet, undereat, or overeat compulsively. Selfish interests are supplanted by interest in others. We do things to benefit others and to benefit society. Here we give the gift that asks no reward.

FOR TODAY: I decide what my attainment markers will be as I go along today.

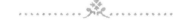

The fertile ground found in Twelve Step Recovery rooms and principles gave me recovery. Now, I give. Conscience prompts me to share my story with others. I have soundness of mind.

The Three Legacies of Twelve Step Programs patterned on A.A. are Recovery, Unity and Service. OA, and other Twelve Step programs rely on these figurative legacies. Personal recovery depends on our helping one another by telling the truth and living according to principles that have been found to be helpful.

"The great thing about getting older is that you don't lose all the other ages you've been." --Madeline L'Engel, Writer

ife is long. The child is in me, the adolescent, the young person, and the person I am now. All these ages are with me in my recovery. I give myself a chance to recover over time. Others see me as I recover over time.

It does not matter what age anyone is. Enter at any point.

"The human spirit rises above the labors of the flesh. The human spirit rises above the transformations of the body. As everyone knows who has truly cared for and loved another, love goes beyond the flesh. It assumes a holy relationship to the other - where changes in the flesh do not go. Changes in the flesh cannot mortify love. Love for another through time sees changes in the flesh, yet it is not daunted." --Judy Briggs, Writer

So it is with recovering people in fellowship over time. Our recoveries go beyond whatever transformations the body may make.

FOR TODAY: Others watch gently as I recover over time. I let myself have this recovery too. I am new today. I will be new tomorrow too, whatever age I'm at.

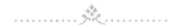

"I am still one of the afflicted. It helps me to remember the sum is greater than the parts." --Anonymous

I am always "one of many." Troubled dieters, overeaters, undereaters, people with substance abuse problems, and behavior addictions come into Twelve Step Recovery programs.

Predecessors built the foundation of recovery. It was through the unconditional love that emanated from the people in Overeaters Anonymous and other Twelve Step rooms that I was able to discard diet substances and compulsive dieting as my Higher Power. My limited purpose to achieve a certain waist size and number on the scale, metamorphosed to another purpose. I want health. I want health for you too. I am no longer satisfied with wishes in a box to achieve love. The great void has been filled.

Gradually new doors open. There is more available to me, and more available of me, than I realized before. The good that is in me is able to express itself. I work with others more easily and contribute to the goodness of their lives.

FOR TODAY: The world is not a dark fearful place.

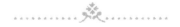

GOING BEYOND THE TERRORS OF LOVE   DECEMBER 20

Committing to love is not so terrifying, or fearing rejection. I don't need to control so much.

FOR TODAY: I do not need to take diet substances or diet compulsively. I go beyond the terrors of love.

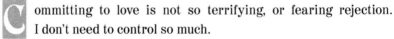

"A happy woman is one who has no cares at all; a cheerful woman is one who has cares, but doesn't let them get her down."
        --Beverly Sills, Opera Singer & Arts Director

"I believe in rainbows and all of that. But there are darker colors . . . and it's the shade that defines the light."
        --Tori Amos, Singer

Many of our heroines could be the star of this opera named "Vanquishing Sadness." Today I live a rich productive satisfying life. I have integrity when I claim my talents.

For Today: Playing the leading role in my life, I am "on" today. I play it with generosity and joy.

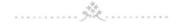

"Before my recovery, I hardly ever laughed. I was so serious. I was so frozen. Since I've come unthawed from receiving love, I laugh. My sweetheart often says he wants to see that smile."
        --Anonymous

"'When you're fat to the point that it's not healthy, there's no humor' –Guest.
How do you get to that point where you are satisfied with your weight?" –Joey Reynolds, WOR Radio Host

For Today: Laughing in the right places and the right spots, lets people know who I am. Making humor lets people know what I find humorous and endearing in life.

"If we are to achieve a richer culture - one rich in contrasting values - we must recognize the whole gamut of human potentialities, and so weave a less arbitrary social fabric, one in which each diverse human gift will find a fitting place."
                    --Margaret Mead, Anthropologist

"Why should an Oak aspire to be a Maple. Or a Maple aspire to be an Oak?" --Anonymous

"To have the sense of one's own intrinsic worth which constitutes self-respect is potentially to have everything; the ability to discriminate, to love and to remain indifferent. To lack it is to be locked within oneself, paradoxically incapable of either love or indifference." --Joan Didion, Writer

"Truth is in our individual worth and dignity. We gain strength because we are together in infinite variety and mesh our various and different qualities." --Kenneth O. Jones, Minister & Writer

"We all have different genes. Our genes behave differently."
                    --Hillary Rodham Clinton, U.S. Secretary of State

The "indifference" Joan Didion refers to, the monk Thomas Merton similarly refers to as "disinterested activity." It is the freedom from self-consciousness and self-absorption, and absorption with other people. It is partly freedom from the distractions of variety, or having to categorize such variety and put value judgments on it. It is the freedom from these disturbances to carry on one's life with joy and enthusiasm and to have self-directed purpose.

We are not trapped by our size or shape or our genes. Variety in faces, skin, hairtones, eyes, mouths, noses, shoulders, waist and hip shapes, heights, legs, breast, bosom, chest, feet, shows diversity in human beings – formations and abilities.

We may be trapped by our attitudes – but Twelve Step Recovery shows how we can become aware of our attitudes and build on identity.

Instead of chasing figments or fantasies, or bemoaning and complaining, I can develop my human potential and what wonderful thing I can do. I can change my perspective. I can have a sense of my own value, and value my body, health, and God-given talents, abilities and enthusiasms.

I am relieved of the deadly compulsions regarding food and dieting. 'Alcoholic thinking', 'diethead thinking,' 'body criticism thinking' are all forms of 'stinking thinking.' They do not build up. Love builds up. Living up to my Purpose, contributing to Life and Creation, builds up.

FOR TODAY: I won't try to fit in the wrong size shoes. They would pinch or flop around. I walk in shoes that fit me. I am glad for me. I am glad for you. Diversity in nature is. I am a living flesh and blood, thinking, perceiving, feeling human being.

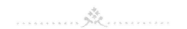

Love may be rejected when offered, may be abused, may be ridiculed as weakness, but love can never, never be destroyed. As I build on identity I am willing to give up my infantile hurts and bitterness as I think about love. I love. Whether I am loved in return does not detract from my love. My love means I have something of value to give.

This doesn't mean I deny the existence of people who cheat. I still have the ability to take care of myself and love.

When I give a gift, and select it carefully, and give from my heart, there is no asking that I get a reward or that the other person gives back. That is why it is a gift. It is a self-gift.

I have only so many days and so many breaths on this earth. So why should I manipulate or calculate who is one up. *"How many angels can dance on the head of a pin,"* is a favorite quotation to question and express skepticism in measurement. The skeptic who said this offers us also an openness to discard measurement too. Measurement after all is a human creation, a tool of the human mind. We can choose to act right, to give love, to mind, regardless of whether anyone is "looking," or whether we will be rewarded or noticed.

"Tensions may be relieved and hearts attuned to be receptive to healing, forgiveness, grace, and love." --Kenneth O. Jones. Fellowship is restoring.

For Today: Helping another person is a gift that asks no reward.

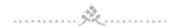

"In singing rehearsal at first - the first sight reading sounds discordant, not like music at all. We stumble. The stronger ones, the section leaders, carry the right notes. They have the melody and sense of forward movement. Some of us, like me have intuitive rhythm but not assurance at first. On the second sing through, and the third, it begins to sound like music, not notes. By the time we get to the performance we are really putting out, putting it all together. We are also listening to one another – to the strong assured leaders. We are performing 'music.'" –Anonymous

"Listen to one another. If you can't hear the person next to you, you are singing too loud." –Music Director

The music of joy comes as we stumble through recovery. We put the pieces together. We learn to listen. We learn to hear one another. We are relieved of the deadly compulsions regarding food and dieting we have been smitten with.

FOR TODAY: I hear the music. It comes from the steps of the practice.

STEADYING STRENGTH COMES   DECEMBER 26

"Being alive, living in abstinence, I see a steadying strength. It reaches me. Others help me. I have strong bonds." --Anonymous

Steadying strength comes. If I get discouraged, it is a sign my resources are depleted. I have gotten too Hungry – Angry – Lonely or Tired (H.A.L.T.). Moreover, it is a reminder that I have wandered back over into self-centered territory: "I am the center of the Universe." "I am responsible for everything about my physical self, spirit and matter." "I have to do it all." This is E.G.O. – Easing God Out. It is good to be alive and healthy!

FOR TODAY: I appreciate what is given. I have strong bonds, feeling these strong bonds, even in silence and when there is distance.

"Silence is the perfectest herald of joy: I were but little happy, if I could say how much."
    –William Shakespeare, *Much Ado About Nothing*

"I am happy as a clam." –Sister to Brother
"I am happy as a clam." –Brother to Sister
Conversation at Wedding Rehearsal Dinner
    --Anonymous

Without fanfare, happiness comes quietly. Going with the flow of life, trusting my mobility to move toward something good, because it is intended for me and I choose it, I obey the spiritual laws of existence. Instead of demanding people, places, and things make me happy, I ask God for acceptance and self-acceptance. Living on the basis of "unsatisfied demands", or disregard for how I am made, is foolish. Abundant nourishing life comes to me,

I dedicate myself to 'this good' - what I have chosen. Dedicating myself to 'this good' affirms it a good, and I have chosen it. It may come to the exclusion of other goods. Living in this awareness, I am not all over the place. When tempted to be jealous of other people's good, I remember - I dedicate myself to 'this good.' My life will have happiness as my one and only life.

In making my ethical choices, I like myself more. The more I like myself, the more I want to make good food choices. The less the "mental blank spot" talked about in *The A.A. Big Book* creeps in. I am relieved a day at a time of the insane urge I was smitten with to diet compulsively, or to overeat and or undereat. Happiness comes when I offer my smile and caring words. I understand another troubled overeater. We are not in a contest, locked in our armor.

FOR TODAY: I open up. I let life come to me. I feel the joy of living.

"It is a design for living that works in rough going."
--Alcoholics Anonymous, Third Edition

"After being abstinent for many years, I wondered if Twelve Step Recovery would work when the going got tough. The World Trade Center got bombed in my City, I had to fly to Hawaii to my neice's wedding, I lost my brother to an accident two days after the wedding, and my sweetheart died -- and all this happened in a short period. The principles I had learned years earlier in OA gave me courage. Members in fellowship helped. I was not overwhelmed. The joy of living is continuing to grow."
--Anonymous

he *A.A. Twelve Steps & Twelve Traditions* talks about difficult times. Would we be up to the task of holding on to our abstinence? Would we be able to refrain from compulsive overeating or using and practicing methods of compulsive dieting? *"...in times of war?"* War may be a metaphor for especially troubled times. It may be a metaphor for our battle with our own thoughts, flights of desire, desire to escape the moment, changes in body size shape and weight.

FOR TODAY: The joy of living is in continuing to grow.

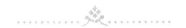

My freedom is the freedom to not have to take a diet remedy or compulsively overeat today. I also have the freedom of acceptance, the freedom to reduce grandiosity and expectations, and to be relieved of the burden of self.

FOR TODAY: Centered balance feels good.

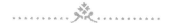

"Move one grain of sand on the beach, and the whole beach changes." –Author Unknown

Being happy, joyous and free has a lot to do with my perception of myself and my relatedness to others. Today I move one grain of sand on the beach, to keep this perception positive and my relatedness right.

FOR TODAY: I know how to move one grain of sand. Small adjustments keep me happy. Am I warm enough? Do I have enough to eat and the right things to eat? Can I help where I didn't think I wanted to help, by doing one small thing?

olding on and letting go is the natural reflex of the heart muscle and valves, the hands, the mouth of the suckling babe. It is the order of the seasons - one season yields to the next. It is the order of the days. Night yields to day. The earth yields and moves.

As the year comes to an end, I can let go of the old insanity. I can let go of my old self, confident there is a new skin. There will be a new look to the New Year. I have the memory of the old. I decide what to leave in the past, and what to take as my balance brought forward . My ledger is full and there are good things to be carried into the New Year.

I have had a good year. I list accomplishments. I list five things I did well. I list main losses and hurts. I acknowledge them. I will not shut the door on them. Nor will I dwell on them.

FOR TODAY: I make a list of a few goals for the New Year! Foremost, will be my commitment to be abstinent and to continue to work on my recovery by working the Twelve Steps of Alcoholics Anonymous and Overeaters Anonymous. This commitment gives me assurance. I won't be starting on a new insanity. The only thing God asks of me is to do the best I can.

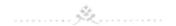

INDEX

Courage, Courageous Jan. 1, Jan. 6, Jan. 23, Mar. 17, Apr. 5, May. 21, June. 20, June. 29, July. 26, Aug. 27, Aug. 31, Sept. 9, Sept. 29, Sept. 30, Oct. 3, Oct. 6, Oct. 11, Oct. 21, Oct. 23, Nov. 25, Dec. 28

Courtesy Nov. 29

Cover-Up Feb. 3, Mar. 21

Covet Feb. 9

Crashing Jan. 3

Crave Sept. 17

Crazy (See Insanity) July. 6

Creation, Create, Co-Create, Created World, Creating Jan. 26, Feb. 10, Mar. 23, Mar. 29, Apr. 10, Apr. 29, May. 15, June. 5, June. 20, July. 8, Aug. 7, Aug. 11, Aug. 20, Sept. 22, Oct. 3, Oct. 16, Oct. 20, Oct. 21, Oct. 24, Oct. 31, Dec. 23

Creating Problems June 5

Creating Safe Boundaries Sept 22

Creation; Co-Creation (See Creation)

Creativity (See Creation)

Creator (See Creation)

Crisis May. 27, June. 8

Critic, Critical Apr. 8, June. 9, Aug. 5, Aug. 17, Sept. 16

Criticism, Criticize Critic, Critical Mar. 20, Mar. 22, Mar. 23, Apr. 8, June. 9, July. 19, Aug. 4, Aug. 5, Aug. 17, Aug. 27, Sept. 16, Nov. 26, Nov. 28

Cruelty, Cruel, Cruella deVille Jan. 18, Jan. 19, Jan. 20, Mar. 15, July. 15, Aug. 7

Culture Feb. 28, Mar. 15, Mar. 17, Oct. 18, Nov. 29

Curb Jan. 7, Mar. 11, Apr. 13, May. 10, June. 5

Cynicism July. 8, Oct. 30

Damage Aug. 29, Aug. 31

Dancing To The Tune Apr. 8

Danger, Dangers Jan. 6, Jan. 16, Apr. 7, Apr. 9, Apr. 13, Apr. 15, Apr. 24, Apr. 25, Oct. 6

Daring Adventure Jan. 16

Darkness, Dark Jan. 30, Mar. 29, Aug. 26

Date Jan. 5

Daunting Aug. 20

Davis, Adele Dec. 8

Daydreams Oct. 12, Oct. 16

Dealing With Disappointment Feb. 22

Dealing With Others Sept. 23

Death Feb. 12, Apr. 15, May. 23, Oct. 25

Debate Sept. 16

Deciding For Ourselves June 4

Deciding My Balance With Love & Sex

Decisions,Decision-Making (See Choices, Decisions)

Deception, Deceitful, Deceive May. 1, May. 13, May. 14, May. 16, May. 17, May. 26, Aug. 1, Aug. 13

Deceiving Myself May 16

Deceiving Ourselves May 17

Deciding My Balance With Love & Sex (See Choices, Decisions, Love, Sex) Aug 14

Defeat, Defeated, Defeatism Feb. 22, July. 2, July. 29

Defect, Defects July. 29, Aug. 2, Aug. 5, Aug. 6, Aug. 9, Aug. 10, Aug. 12, Aug. 20, Aug. 21

Defense, Defending, Defensive, Defense Mechanisms Feb. 3, Mar. 18, June. 20, Aug. 27, Sept. 1

Defiance Mar. 9

Definition, Define, Defining May. 6, May. 7, June 30

Defining A Lie May 1-31

Defining New Terms For Success Feb. 23, Feb. 24, Mar. 1, Apr. 17, Apr. 26, May. 6-8, June. 6, July. 3, Sept. 17, Oct. 12, Oct. 15, Oct. 29, Dec. 2

Defining The Difference (See Definition) June 30

Dejection Aug. 22

Delay Oct. 18

Deliberation Oct. 21

Delight Sept. 10, Oct. 19, Nov. 20

Delirium Apr. 23, Apr. 24

Delusion July. 2

Demand, Demanding, Demands, Unsatisfied Demands Jan. 16, Aug. 13, Aug. 17, Aug. 23, Aug. 24, Aug. 26, Oct. 7

Demanding Of Protection (See Demand)

Demeaning Apr. 28

Demoralizing, Demoralized Jan. 25, Mar. 6

Denial, Deny Feb. 1, May. 2, Aug. 9, Aug. 10, Aug. 11, Aug. 13, Aug. 20, Aug. 25, Aug. 27, Aug. 31, Sept. 11, Sept. 19, Oct. 27, Dec. 24

Dependence, Dependent Jan. 16, Oct. 14, Nov. 8, Dec. 9

Dependence On Others (See Dependence)

Depletion, Depleted Feb. 27

Depression Feb. 22, Aug. 11, Nov. 26

Deprivation Aug. 13, Oct. 15, Nov. 28

De-Self, De-Selfing (See Self, Self-Abnegation, Self-Absorption, Self-Acceptance, Self-Care, Self-Centered, Self-Concept, Self-Condemnation, Self-Criticism, Self-Deception, Self-Defense, Self-Defined, Self-Denying, Self-Destructive, Self-Dissatisfaction, Self-Driven Health, Self-Effacing, Self-Enhancement, Self-Esteem, Self-Loathing, Self-Knowledge, Self-Pity, Self-Punishment, Self-Regard, Self-Respect, Self-Seeking, Self-Will, Self-Worth, De-Self)

Design Feb. 10

Desire, Desires, Desirable Feb. 1, Feb. 11, Mar. 25, Apr. 4, Apr. 17, June. 16, June. 26, July. 30, Aug. 1, Aug. 13, Aug. 20, Aug. 26, Aug. 27, Sept. 18, Oct. 16, Oct. 20

Despair, Despairing, Despondent Jan. 25, Jan. 27, Feb. 16, Apr. 5, May. 23, June. 12, June. 17, June. 20, July. 7, July. 8, July. 20, Aug. 2, Aug. 11, Aug. 17, Aug. 22, Sept. 4, Sept. 13, Oct. 30, Nov. 19, Dec. 7

Desperation, Desperate Jan. 1, Jan. 2, Jan. 3, Jan. 5, Jan. 19, Jan. 20, Jan. 28, Jan. 29, Jan. 30, Feb. 3, Mar. 1, Apr. 4, Apr. 5, Apr. 27, June. 11, June. 15, June. 16, Aug. 13, Nov. 12, Nov. 30, Dec. 10, Dec. 11, Dec. 15

Despondent Jan. 25

Destroy, Destruction Mar. 17 July. 2, July. 8, Aug. 5, Aug. 7, Aug. 26

Detach, Detaching Jan. 19, May. 12, Sept. 20, Oct. 15

Detaching From Erroneous Messages Sept. 20

Detractor Feb. 24

Develop July. 13, Oct. 16, Oct. 17, Oct. 19

Diderot, Denis Aug. 17, Sept. 10

Didion, Joan May. 17, June. 26, Dec. 23

Diethead, Diet Head (See Stinking Thinking) Mar 13, Dec. 23

INDEX

ACKNOWLEDGEMENTS & PERMISSIONS

Quotations by individual authors and editions are reprinted under fair use copyright permission.

Authors' writings are available in libraries and from www.amazon.com and other fine bookstores.
Kenneth O. Jones, *Lean Back on the Everlasting Arms* is currently available by writing to Fifth Avenue Presbyterian Church, 7 Fifth Avenue, N.Y., N.Y. 10007, www.fapc.org.

Recovering Compulsive Dieter - Daily Meditations is also published under the title *Letting Go of Diet Remedies-Twelve Step Recovery From Use of Diet Substances & Compulsive Dieting.*

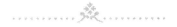

LaVergne, TN USA
12 October 2009
160567LV00005B/15/P